The Adult with Tetralogy of Fallot

The ISACCD Monograph Series

Edited by

Michael A. Gatzoulis, MD, PhD, FACC

Director, Adult Congenital Heart Programme,
Royal Brompton Hospital, London, UK

and

Daniel J. Murphy, Jr., MD, FACC

Staff Cardiologist, The Center for Pediatric
and Congenital Heart Diseases,
The Cleveland Clinic Foundation, Ohio, US

Futura Publishing Company, Inc.
Armonk, NY 2001

Library of Congress Cataloging-in-Publication Data

The adult with tetralogy of Fallot / edited by Michael A. Gatzoulis & Daniel
J. Murphy, Jr.
    p. ; cm.
    Includes bibliographical references and index.
    ISBN 0-87993-490-5 (alk. paper)
    1. Tetralogy of Fallot. I. Gatzoulis, Michael A. II. Murphy, Daniel J., Jr.
    [DNLM: 1. Tetralogy of Fallot. WG 220 A2449 2001]
  RC687 .A46 2001
  616.1′2043–dc21

                               2001023865

Every effort has been made to ensure that the information in this book is
as up to date and accurate as possible at the time of publication. However,
due to the constant developments in medicine, neither the author, nor the
editor, nor the publisher can accept any legal or any other responsibility
for any errors or omissions that may occur.

Printed in the United States of American on acid-free paper.

Contents

Foreword

This monograph is the first of a series dedicated to common topics in adult congenital heart disease (CHD). Co-sponsored by the International Society of Adult Congenital Cardiac Disease (ISACCD) and Futura Media Services, this series will provide comprehensive, timely reviews of the major forms of CHD in the adult. The authors are internationally renowned experts, actively involved in research into the clinical problems facing this patient population. This project arose from scientific presentations at the biannual ISACCD meetings, which although invaluable to the audience in attendance, will have a much greater impact reaching the broader community of professionals practicing in the field.

The chapters in this monograph contain background information and current data on the major clinical problems which face adults with tetralogy of Fallot (TOF). Each monograph is intended as both an introduction to the subject and a timely, comprehensive review, more extensive than a review article and more up-to-date than a textbook. As such, this monograph should be of interest to internists, cardiologists, pediatric cardiologists, and surgeons who finds theselves encountering adults with congenital heart defects with increasing frequency in practice. It should also be useful to trainees, nurses and other professionals as an introduction to the topic of TOF in the adult. Key references provided at the end of each chapter identifies the relevant literature on the subject and allows for further reading.

The reader will detect a consistent theme as individual authors discuss different long-term problems facing this patient population; this is theme is the limited scientific information upon which to base management recommendations. Rather than providing a "cookbook" for care of the adult with TOF, therefore, this monograph will serve as a stimulus for generating key therapeutic questions and, it is hoped, research projects necessary to answer them. The adult who was born with TOF, although "fixed" is not "cured." Improving survival and quality of life for this growing adult population will continue to challenge the current and future generations of congenital cardiologists.

The editors are grateful for the excellent and timely contributions of the authors who have shared their clinical and research experience with us. We also gratefully acknowledge the assistance of Jacques Strauss, President, Futura Publishing Co. who has been a generous, enthusiastic supporter of this project from its inception. Finally, this monograph would not have been possible without the foresight and leadership of the founders and officers of the ISACCD.

Daniel J. Murphy, Jr., MD
President, ISACCD

Michael A. Gatzoulis, MD, PhD, FACC
Secretary, ISACCD

Contributors

Seshadri Balaji, MBBS, MRCP, FACC   Adjunct Associate Professor, Department of Pediatrics, Division of Cardiology and Director, Pediatric Arrhythmias, Pacing and Electrophysiology, Oregon Health Sciences, Portland, Oregon, USA

Andrew D., Blaufox MD, FACC   Assistant Professor of Pediatrics, Staff Pediatric Cardiologist, The Children's Heart Program of South Carolina, MUSAC, Charleston, South Carolina, USA

Derize Boshoff, MD   Senior Fellow, Department of Pediatric and Congenital Cardiology University Hospital Gasthuisberg, Leuven, Belgium

Eugene Downer, MD   Professor of Medicine, Electrophysiologist, University of Toronto Congenital Cardiac Centre for Adults, Toronto General Hospital/University Health Network, Toronto, Ontario, Canada

Michael A. Gatzoulis, MD, PhD, FACC   Director, Adult Congenital Heart Program, Consultant Cardiologist, Royal Brompton Hospital & Senior Lecturer, National Heart & Lung Institute, London, UK

Marc H. Gewillig, MD, PhD, FACC   Professor, Director of Pediatric Cardiology, Department of Pediatric and Congenital Cardiology, University Hospital Gasthuisberg, Leuven, Belgium

Paul G. Gillette, MD   Professor of Pediatrics, Director, Cook Children's Arrhythmia Center, Fort Worth, Texas, USA

Thomas P. Graham Jr., MD, FACC   Ann & Monroe Carell Family Professor of Pediatrics, Director, Pediatric Cardiology, Vanderbilt University Medical Center, Nashville, Tennessee, USA

Louise Harris, MB,ChB, FRCP (C), FACC   Associate Professor of Medicine, Electrophysiologist, University of Toronto Congenital Cardiac Centre for Adults, Toronto General Hospital/University Health Network, Toronto, Ontario, Canada

John S. Hokanson, MD   Staff Paediatric Cardiologist, Children's Hospital of Illinois, University of Illinois College of Medicine, Peoria, Illinois, USA

Peter R. McLaughlin, MD, FRCP(C), FACC   Professor of Medicine, University of Toronto, Staff Cardiologist, University of Toronto Congenital Cardiac Centre for Adults, University Health Network, Toronto, Ontario, Canada

James H. Moller, MD, FACC   Professor of Pediatrics, Director, Pediatric Cardiology, University of Minnesota, Minneapolis, Minnesota, USA

Makoto Nakazawa, MD   Professor, Department of Pediatric Cardiology, The Heart Institute of Japan, Tokyo Women's Medical University, Tokyo, Japan

Andrew N. Redington, MD, MRCP   Professor of Congenital Heart Disease, Great Ormond Street Hospital, London, UK

Tony M. Reybrouck, PhD   Professor, Director of Pediatric Exercise Physiology Laboratory, Department of Paediatric and Congenital Cardiology, University Hospital Gasthuisberg, Leuven, Belgium

Philip J. Saul, MD   Professor of Pediatrics, Chief of Pediatric Cardiology, The Children's Heart Program of South Carolina, MUSAC, Charleston, South Carolina, USA

Tokuko Shinohara, MD   Staff Cardiologist, Department of Paediatric Cardiology, Heart Institute of Japan Tokyo Women's Medical University, Tokyo, Japan

Samuel C. Siu, MD, FRCP(C), FACC   Assistant Professor of Medicine, Staff Cardiologist, Toronto General Hospital/University Health Network, Director of Research, University of Toronto Congenital Cardiac Centre for Adults, Toronto, Ontario, Canada

Glen S. Van Arsdell, MD   Assistant Professor, Staff Cardiologist Cardiovascular Surgery, The Hospital for Sick Children and Toronto General Hospital, University of Toronto, Toronto, Ontario, Canada

Gary D. Webb, MD, FRCP(C), FACC   Bitove Professor of Adult Congenital Heart Disease, Director, University of Toronto Congenital Cardiac Centre for Adults, Member, Heart and Stroke/Richard Lewar Centre of Excellence, University of Toronto, Division of Cardiology, Toronto General Hospital, Professor of Medicine, University of Toronto, Toronto, Ontario, Canada

Steven A. Webber, MBCHB, FACC   Associate Professor of Medicine, University of Pittsburgh School of Medicine, Pittsburgh, Pennsylvania, USA

William G. Williams, MD, FRCS(C)   Professor and Head, Cardiovascular Surgery, The Hospital for Sick Children and Toronto General Hospital, University of Toronto, Toronto, Ontario, Canada

Chapter I

Risk Stratification for Arrhythmia and Sudden Cardiac Death Late after Repair of Tetralogy of Fallot

Michael A. Gatzoulis,
Seshadri Balaji, Steven A. Webber,
Samuel C. Siu, John S. Hokanson,
Tokuko Shinohara, Makoto Nakazawa,
James H. Moller, Paul C. Gillette,
Gary D. Webb, Andrew N. Redington

Introduction

Intracardiac repair for tetralogy of Fallot, the most common cyanotic congenital heart disease, has been performed for over 4 decades.[1-3] Although early and long-term results of repair are excellent, clinical arrhythmia and sudden cardiac death remain problematic.[3-7] The latter has been consistently reported in all follow-up series and constitutes the largest single cause of late mortality associated with repaired tetralogy.[8] There is some evidence to suggest a cause-and-effect relationship between arrhythmia and sudden death in these patients.[9,10] However, the pathogenic mechanism of sudden death remains unclear.

Even if the optimism that modifications of surgical protocols will reduce the incidence of late complications is realized,[11] large numbers of adult patients who underwent tetralogy repair in a previous era are currently followed in outpatient clinics. These patients represent a challenge to physicians involved with their care, particularly in terms of risk stratification for arrhythmia and sudden death.[12,13] We,[14,15] and oth-

From Gatzoulis MA, Murphy DJ (eds): *The Adult with Tetralogy of Fallot: The ISACCD Monograph Series* ©Futura Publishing Co., Inc, Armonk, NY, 2001.

ers,[16,17] have recently shown that simple electrocardiographic markers are related to these devastating late complications in single center cohorts of late follow-up patients with repaired tetralogy. In this study, we examined these markers[18] and the potential important characteristics[12] in a large cohort of patients operated upon in several centers, by many different surgeons. Our aim was to validate and refine risk stratification for clinical arrhythmia and sudden death and attempt to shed light in the pathogenesis of these phenomena following repair of tetralogy.

Methods

We identified from hospital databases and recorded the available 10-year records (1985–1995) of all patients with tetralogy of Fallot alive in 1985 (following previous repair) who were followed up periodically at the six participating centers until 1995 (or the occurrence of death). We excluded patients with coexistent atrioventricular septal defect, double outlet right ventriculo-arterial connection, absent pulmonary valve syndrome, those with aorto-pulmonary window, patients requiring a conduit repair and patients with major extracardiac/chromosomal abnormalities. We also excluded patients who received a pacemaker for post-operative complete heart block, and patients who developed clinical arrhythmias prior to 1985.

Detailed surgical history, including the type of right ventricular (RV) outflow reconstruction, was obtained from operative notes. The follow-up status of the patients was determined from the hospital records and clinic visits. If a clinical review had not been performed within 12 months of the 1995 inclusion date, contact with primary physicians and/or patients was made. Clinical arrhythmia, in the form of sustained atrial flutter/fibrillation or ventricular tachycardia (VT) and sudden death were the primary endpoints of the study. The arrhythmia group comprised all patients who presented between 1985–1995 with either 1) sustained, symptomatic atrial flutter/fibrillation (paroxysmal or chronic) or sustained monomorphic VT documented by a 12 lead-electrocardiogram (ECG) or Holter recording, or 2) palpitations associated with near syncope or syncope, subsequently found to have sustained atrial flutter/fibrillation or monomorphic VT at electrophysiological testing. Sustained was defined as arrhythmia lasting >30 sec, or of any time-length if associated with symptoms. Patients with non-sustained runs of atrial or ventricular arrhythmia on Holter monitoring were not included in the arrhythmia group. Other events, such as re-operations and non-sudden cardiac death were also recorded. Electrocardiogram parameters (QRS duration, dispersion of QT, RR interval, superior QRS axis [$-180°$ to $0°$] and the presence of U wave) were analyzed manually from standard (25 mm/s speed and 1 mV/cm standardization) resting 12-lead sinus electrocardiograms as previously described.[14,15,19–21] QRS duration was defined as the maximal QRS length in any lead from the first to the final sharp vector crossing the isoelectric line.[14] U waves were included in the analysis when prominent (U wave ≥ 50% of T wave) or biphasic. The dispersion of QT was measured only in patients with clinical endpoints and/or a QRS duration of 160 ms or greater.[15] Rate of QRS change was taken as the absolute change in QRS duration divided by the number of intervening years (1985 to 1995 or the year of clinical arrhythmia or sudden death). ECG parameters from patients started on antiarrhythmic drugs or drugs known to affect QRS complex and the QT interval were not included in the analysis. Cardiothoracic ratio from the postero-anterior chest radiograph was used as an estimate of cardiac size. The available echocardiograms were recorded using many different commercially available machines, and by many different operators, making detailed analysis impossible. Nonetheless, the presence of residual ventricular septal defect, the RV systolic pressure (estimated from tricuspid regurgitation velocities, assuming a right atrial pressure of 10 mmHg), RV outflow tract peak instantaneous systolic gradient, the right-to-left ventricular end-diastolic diameter from M-mode parasternal long-axis views, and the subjective severity of tricuspid and pulmonary regurgitation (graded: absent or mild, moderate and severe) were recorded when available. Right ventricular systolic and end-diastolic pressure, right-to-left ventricular pressure ratios and the presence of peripheral pulmonary artery stenosis (thought to be hemodynamically important) at cardiac catheterization were all recorded. Standard Holter recordings obtained with a Tracker (Reynolds, UK), Cardiodata PR3 (Milwaukee, WI), or Oxford MR4 (Oxford Instruments Inc. Medical Systems Div., Clearwater, FL) monitor systems were analyzed using the Cardiodata Mark 4 system, Oxford Excel or Marquette Electronics SXP Analysis System (Marquette Medical Systems, Milwaukee, WI). Modified Lown criteria,[22] according to Deanfield et al[23] were used to grade the frequency and complexity of ventricular arrhythmia during 24-hour monitoring. Where multiple Holter recordings per patient were available, the highest Lown grade within the study period and prior to onset of arrhythmia was used for the analysis. Electrophysiological studies were performed primarily for investigation of symptoms (palpitations or presyncope/syncope) but not in all patients with arrhythmia or symptoms due to different local practices. During electrophysiologic testing, ventricular stimulation was performed in all patients and included two extrastimuli at two or three sites at two rates.[24] Inducibility of sustained monomorphic VT, and point of origin (apex, infundibulum, or both) were recorded in all.

ECG data were recorded from 1985 (entry year) and 1995 (exit year/if patient alive); when primary events (clinical arrhythmia and sudden death) occurred, additional ECG data were recorded from the year preceding the event. Available echocardiographic and cardiac catheterization data obtained during the preceding 12 months from the last patient assessment in 1995 or prior to the occurrence of clinical arrhythmia or sudden death were also recorded. Finally, we recorded all electrophysiological studies prior to reinterventions and all reinterventions occurring at any stage during the study.

For statistical analysis we classified patients in four subgroups: patients with sustained VT, sudden death, atrial flutter/fibrillation and the remainder (arrhythmia-free group). Patients with two or more primary endpoints were classified according to the latest event, i.e., a patient with previous VT dying suddenly was classified as a sudden death case. Data were collected locally, whereas final analysis was performed centrally. Inter and intra-observer variability was tested on a random sample of 15 ECGs from each participating center, analyzed by two blinded investigators.

Data Analysis

Data analysis was performed using SPSS for Windows software (Version 7.5). Descriptive data for continuous variables are presented as mean ± standard deviation (SD) or median with range when appropriate. Chi-square or Fisher's exact tests were used to compare discrete variables. Data were analyzed across the four subgroups with Kruskal Wallis and, where a significant difference was found, were further investigated with paired Student's t or Wilcoxon rank-sum test; adjustments were made for multiple comparisons ($p = 0.05/6 = 0.008$). Patients were classified according to the latest clinical event in cases of overlap between primary end-points. Linear regression analysis between QRS duration and cardiothoracic ratio was performed. The probability of remaining free of clinical arrhythmia or sudden death over time was displayed using Kaplan-Meier plots. Univariate analysis of predictors of VT, sudden death and atrial flutter/fibrillation was performed using Cox's proportional hazard model. Predictors for each outcome were analyzed separately. Univariate predictors with a significant level of < 0.10 were entered into a multivariate Cox's proportional hazard model utilizing a backwards elimination algorithm.[25] The level of significance for the multivariate model was set at 0.05. Collinearity between univariate predictors were assessed; highly correlated predictors (correlation coefficient > 0.70) were combined into a composite variable. A secondary analysis was performed utilizing available longitudinal electrocardiographic (n = 471) and echocardiographic (n = 456) data.

Results

Patients

Seven hundred ninety-three patients (470 males, 323 females) with repaired tetralogy fulfilled entry criteria, allowing for over 7,500 patient-years of follow-up. Their mean age in 1985 was 17.5 ± 10.7 (median 15, range 1.5–72) years. Tetralogy repair had been performed at a mean of 8.2 ± 8 (median 5.7, range 0.2–64.5) years. Repair via the right ventricle was performed in 91%, whereas a transatrial/transpulmonary approach was used for the remainder. Total follow-up time from repair to 1995 (or the time the primary end-point occurred) was a mean of 21.1 ± 8.7 (median 21, 8–41) years, with no significant differences between the four patient subgroups. Most patients (649, or 81.8%) were in NYHA functional class I; 121 (15.3%) were in class II, and 23 (2.9%) in class III. As noted previously, 9 additional patients who had a pacemaker for complete atrioventricular block and 2 patients with episodes of sustained ventricular tachychardia prior to 1985 were excluded. We also excluded 14 (1.7%) patients in whom we were unable to determine current status; information from Death Registries indicated that 12 of them were alive in 1997.

Clinical Data (Table 1)

Sustained Ventricular Tachycardia

Thirty-three of the 793 patients (Figure 1) were identified as having one or more episodes of documented VT between 1985–1995. Twenty-seven of them had one or more syncopal episodes requiring cardiopulmonary resuscitation (near-miss sudden death). The remaining 6 patients presented with palpitations and presyncope. The 35-year probability of remaining free of sustained VT was 88.14% (Figure 2a).

Table 1.
Demographic and Surgical Characteristics.

	VT (n=33)	SD (n=16)	AF (n=29)	Arrhythmia-free (n=715)	P
r. age, years	8.4 ± 6.1	17 ± 15.5	17.9 ± 13	7.5 ± 7.5	<0.001
FU, years	21 ± 7.6	22.8 ± 8.5	21.7 ± 7.3	21 ± 7.3	0.835
Male gender	22 (67%)	9 (56%)	20 (69%)	468 (60%)	0.575
Palliation	18 (55%)	6 (38%)	14 (48%)	256 (36%)	0.095
BT Shunt	14 (78%)	6 (100%)	7 (50%)	211 (84%)	0.006
Transvent.	33 (100%)	15 (94%)	27 (93%)	646 (90%)	0.102
TAP r.	19 (58%)	8 (50%)	10 (34%)	237 (33%)	0.039
Re-interv.	7 (21%)	2 (13%)	8 (28%)	80 (11%)	0.023

VT= sustained ventricular tachycardia; SD= sudden death; AF= atrial flutter/fibrillation; Arrhythmia-free= patients who remained free of clinical arrhythmia and sudden death by the end of the study; r.= repair; FU= follow-up from repair; ( )= relative percentages, i.e. for palliation of the total patients, and for BT shunt of the patients who underwent palliations prior to repair; Transven.: transventricular repair [the remainder underwent repair via a transatrial/transpulmonary approach]; TAP= transannular patch uitilized for RVOT reconstruction; Re-interv.= Re-intevention (surgical and/or transcatheter) prior to 1985.

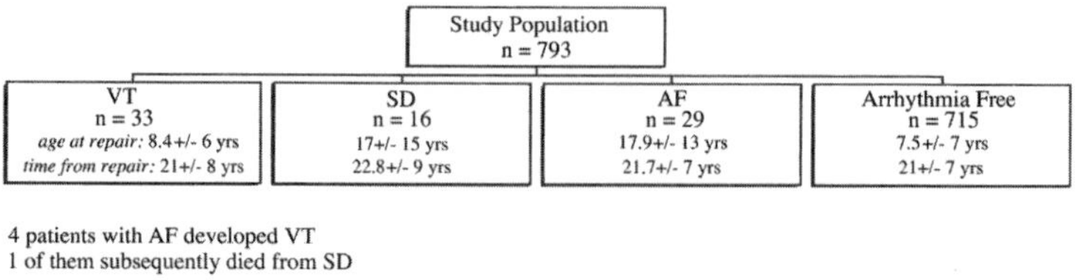

Figure 1. Study population. Note much later repair in patients dying suddenly and those developing atrial flutter/fibrillation during the study, compared to patients with sustained ventricular tachycardia and arrhythmia free.
*Limited overlap between the arrhythmia subgroups and patients who died suddenly.
VT= sustained ventricular tachycardia; SD= sudden cardiac death; AF= atrial flutter/fibrillation; Arrhythmia-free= patients who remained free of clinical arrhythmia and sudden death by the end of the study.

Sudden Death

Sixteen patients died suddenly between 1985–1995. Their mean age was significantly greater than the VT and arrhythmia-free group. Only one of them had previously documented clinical arrhythmia (atrial flutter 3 years prior to death, followed by a syncopal episode due to documented VT 2 years later). Freedom from sudden death over a 35-year period was 91.86% (Figure 2b).

Atrial Flutter/Fibrillation

Twenty-nine patients with one or more episodes of sustained atrial flutter/fibrillation were identified from the total cohort (35-year probability 89.58%, Figure 2c). Their age at repair was significantly greater compared to arrhythmia-free patients and those who developed VT. Their symptoms varied from palpitations (with or without presyncope) in 26 and syncope in 3. Electrical cardioversion was used in 16, whereas the remainder were managed medically. Four patients presenting with atrial flutter/fibrillation developed VT during the study, and are classified in the VT group. Re-interventions for residual hemodynamic problems prior to 1985 were more common in this group (28%).

A transannular patch type of repair was more common in the VT (58%) compared to all other groups ($p = 0.039$, Chi-Square Testing).

There were another 17 deaths during the study period, 12 of which were cardiac (heart failure in 9, re-operation in 1, coronary artery disease

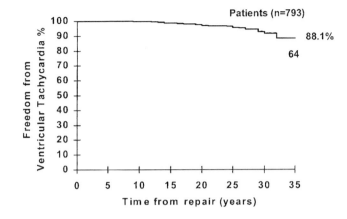

A

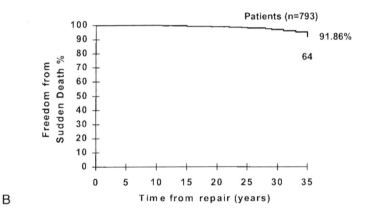

B

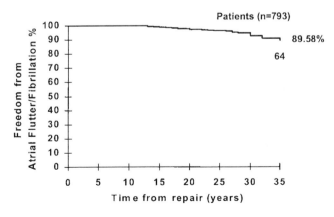

C

Figure 2. Freedom from sustained ventricular tachycardia (2a), sudden cardiac death (2b) and sustained atrial flutter/fibrillation (2c) by Kaplan-Meier survival curves: Total study population.

in 2). The 5 noncardiac deaths were due to accidental causes in 2, Hodgkin's lymphoma in 1, lung cancer in 1 and suicide in 1.

Electrocardiographic & Radiographic Data (Table 2)

Repeated measurements of QRS duration and the dispersion of QT on 90 randomly chosen ECGs were performed twice by the two blinded observers (M.A.G., S.B.). The percentage differences in these measurements for the same ECG ranged from 1% to 8% for within-observer and 2% to 11% for between-observer variability. Maximum QRS ranged between 70 and 240 (mean 151 ± 27, median 155) msecs. QRS duration and the dispersion of QT were prolonged in all 3 primary endpoint groups compared to arrhythmia-free controls (Figure 3). A significantly greater rate of QRS change was observed between 1985 and the year preceding clinical events in the VT and sudden death groups (Figure 4). There were no statistically significant differences between groups in terms of superior QRS axis or U wave on the ECG. There was a weak correlation between QRS and cardiothoracic ratio (CTR) ($r = 0.44$, $p < 0.001$) for the whole group of 793 patients.

Hemodynamic Data (Table 3)

Pulmonary and tricuspid regurgitation with or without peripheral pulmonary artery stenosis were the main residual hemodynamic lesions relating to clinical arrhythmia and sudden death in this study (Figure 5).

Table 2.
Electrocardiographic & Radiographic Data.

	VT (n=31)	SD (n=14)	AF (n=24)	Arrhythmia-free (n=691)	P
RR, ms	826 ± 186	790 ± 235	815 ± 72	797 ± 272	0.738
Superior axis	11 (33%)	5 (31%)	11 (37%)	159 (22%)	0.097
U waves	3 (9%)	1 (6.3%)	6 (20%)	36 (5%)	0.236
QRS, ms	191.5 ± 21	179 ± 24	166.9 ± 21	146.7 ± 24	<0.001
QRS ≥ 180ms	29 (88%)	10 (63%)	10 (34%)	42 (5.9%)	<0.001
QRS ch, ms	4.1 ± 2.2	3.5 ± 1.9	2.1 ± 1.2	1.5 ± 1.2	<0.001
QT d, ms	95.3 ± 28	81.2 ± 25	57.9 ± 32	53.5 ± 22	<0.001
CTR	0.58 ± 0.05	0.63 ± 0.06	0.61 ± 0.05	0.53 ± 0.05	<0.001

VT= sustained ventricular tachycardia; SD= sudden death; AF= atrial flutter/fibrillation; Arrhythmia-free= patients who remained free of clinical arrhythmia and sudden death by the end of the study; RR= RR interval, Superior axis= QRS axis between −180° and 0°; U waves= included when ≥50 of T wave or biphasic; QRS= maximum QRS duration measured manually in any of the 12 leads; QRS ch= Mean change in QRS duration between 1985 and 1995 [or the last ECG prior to onset of arrhythmia or occurrence of sudden death]; QT d= QT dispersion, measured when QRS ≥ 160 ms and/or in patients with clinical end-points on ECGs obtained prior to onset of events.

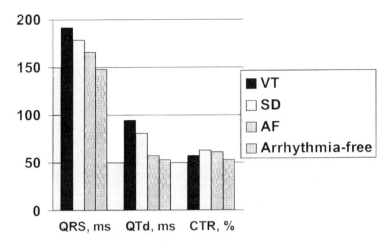

Figure 3. Electrocardiographic and Radiological Data in 793 Patients Late After Repair of Tetralogy of Fallot: Common Electrophysiological Substrate Between Patients with Sustained Ventricular Tachycardia and Sudden Death.

Marked QRS prolongation and QT dispersion in the sustained ventricular tachycardia and sudden death subgroups suggest possible right ventricular dilatation and repolarization abnormalities. Increased cardiothoracic ratios in the ventricular tachycardia, sudden death and atrial flutter/fibrillation groups indicative of impaired hemodynamics (presented data predate the onset of arrhythmia or sudden death).

VT= sustained ventricular tachycardia; SD= sudden cardiac death; AF= atrial flutter/fibrillation; Arrhythmia-free= patients who remained free of clinical arrhythmia and sudden death by the end of the study; CTR= cardiothoracic ratio.

Right ventricular outflow peak instantaneous systolic gradient on Doppler ranged from 0 to 90 mmHg (mean 20.1 ± 5.4, median 16); its severity did not relate to any of the primary endpoints. It was greater than 60 mmHg in 13 and between 35 and 60 mmHg in 27 patients respectively. Tricuspid regurgitation was the predominant lesion within the atrial flutter/fibrillation group, whereas moderate or severe pulmonary regurgitation with or without peripheral pulmonary stenosis was predominant in the group of VT and sudden death.

Holter Data (Table 4)

Holter recordings (single or multiple) were available and reviewed from 346 patients. The frequency and complexity of ventricular arrhythmia—according to the modified Lown criteria[22,23]—was not different in patients with clinical arrhythmia or sudden death, compared to the arrhythmia-free patients. Grade ≥ 2 ventricular arrhythmia on Holter, previously shown to be a risk marker,[26] was not predictive of sudden death in

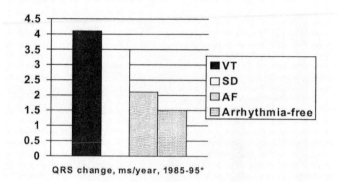

QRS change, ms/year, 1985-95*

Figure 4. Mean Annual QRS Change During the Study*: Different Rates of QRS Prolongation in the 4 Patient Subgroups.

Sustained ventricular tachycardia and sudden death were both preceded by a late, rapid increase in QRS duration, compared to the atrial flutter/fibrillation and arrhythmia-free subgroups, who showed a steady, albeit slower degree of QRS prolongation during the study.

*1985 to 1995 or the year of arrhythmia onset or sudden death.

VT= sustained ventricular tachycardia; SD= sudden cardiac death; AF= atrial flutter/fibrillation; Arrhythmia-free= patients who remained free of clinical arrhythmia and sudden death by the end of the study.

Table 3.
Hemodynamic Data (n=456).

	VT	SD	AF	Arrhythmia-	P free
Echo (n=456)	(n=31)	(n=9)	(n=23)	(n=393)	
Residual VSD	5 (16%)	2 (22%)	4 (17%)	40 (10%)	0.294
RVSP* mmHg	46.1 ± 17.5	50 ± 12.6	41.3 ± 8.8	42.9 ± 18.1	0.589
RVSP > 60 mmHg	5 (16%)	1 (11%)	2 (9%)	46 (12%)	0.636
RVOTO mmHg	15.7 ± 12.2	20.3 ± 6.1	16.1 ± 10.9	19.2 ± 15.4	0.589
RV/LV EDD	1.04 ± 0.31	0.94 ± 0.37	0.79 ± 0.23	0.83 ± 0.31	0.077
TR ≥ moderate	13 (45%)	4 (44%)	16 (70%)	37 (10%)	<0.001
PR ≥ moderate	29 (94%)	9 (100%)	15 (65%)	191 (49%)	<0.001
CC (n=148)	(19)	(2)	(12)	(115)	
RVEDP mmHg	10.3 ± 3.9	9.5 ± 0.7	11.5 ± 3.8	9.4 ± 3.8	0.257
RV/LV pressure	0.39 ± 0.18	0.38 ± 0.11	0.41 ± 0.12	0.44 ± 0.21	0.829
Peripheral PS	8 (42%)	1 (50%)	2 (17%)	18 (15.7%)	0.037

VT= sustained ventricular tachycardia; SD= sudden death; AF= atrial flutter/fibrillation; Arrhythmia-free= patients who remained free of clinical arrhythmia and sudden death by the end of the study; * = assuming right atrial pressure of 10 mmHg; VSD= vetricular septal defect; RVSP= right ventricular systolic pressure; RVOTO= right ventricular outflow tract obstruction; RV/LV EDD= right ventricular/left ventricular end-diastolic diameter, from M-mode parasternal long-axis views; TR= tricuspid regurgitation; PR= pulmonary regurgitation; CC= cardiac catheterization; RVEDP= right ventricular end-diastolic pressure; RV/LV= right ventricular to left ventricular; PS= pulmonary stenosis

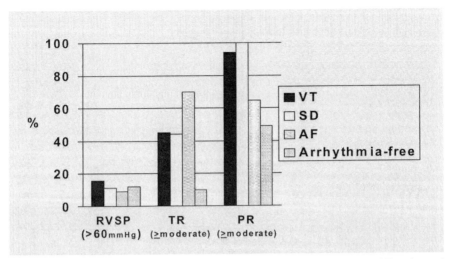

Figure 5. Echocardiographic Data from 456 Patients Late After Repair of Tetralogy of Fallot: Pulmonary Regurgitation is the Culprit Lesion for Sustained Ventricular Tachycardia and Sudden Death.

Lack of difference between the four subgroups in percentage of patients with elevation of systolic right ventricular pressure (> 60 mmHg), suggesting that residual right ventricular outflow obstruction—in isolation—is not responsible for arrhythmia or sudden death late after tetralogy repair. High prevalence of moderate or severe tricuspid and pulmonary regurgitation in the atrial flutter/fibrillation and ventricular tachycardia/sudden death subgroups respectively, indicative of a relationship between specific late hemodynamic substrates and arrhythmia and sudden death.

VT= sustained ventricular tachycardia; SD= sudden cardiac death; AF= atrial flutter/fibrillation; Arrhythmia-free= patients who remained free of clinical arrhythmia and sudden death by the end of the study; RVSP= right ventricular systolic pressure; TR= tricuspid regurgitation; PR= pulmonary regurgitation (please see methods).

this cohort. Furthermore, there was no correlation between asymptomatic runs of VT on Holter recordings (> 3 consecutive ventricular contractions with a mean rate of > 110 beats/min) and the subsequent development of clinical VT ($p = 0.495$, Chi Square test).

Electrophysiological Data (Table 5)

Ninety-one patients with a mean age of 24 ± 11.2 (median 21, range 5–50) years underwent electrophysiological study at 17.4 ± 7.8 (median 17, range 4–39) years from repair and prior to intervention; indications were investigation of symptoms (88%) and/or Holter ventricular arrhythmia (6%), "routine" follow-up protocols (4%), and ablation of previously documented VT (2%). Sustained monomorphic VT was inducible in 32 patients (35%), with hemodynamic compromise in all. The arrhythmia fo-

Table 4.
Holter Data (n=346).

	VT (n=25)	SD (n=6)	AF (n=22)	Arrhythmia-free (n=293)	P *
Lown Criteria†					
0: No ectopy	2	–	2	29	0.54
I: <30/hr, unif.	7	3	5	117	
II: >30/hr, unif.	6	1	10	62	
III: couplets or multif.<30/hr	7	2	4	45	
IV: couplets or multif.>30/hr	2	–	1	32	
V: VT‡	1	–	–	8	
Lown VT = > II	16	3	15	137	0.247

VT= sustained ventricular tachycardia; SD= sudden death; AF= atrial flutter/fibrillation; Arrhythmia-free= patients who remained free of clinical arrhythmia and sudden death by the end of the study; * = chi square test; † = ventricular ectopy according to the modified Lown Criteria; unif.= uniform ventricular extrasystoles; multif.= multiform ventricular extrasystoles; ‡ = >3 consecutive ventricular contractions with a mean rate of >110 beats/min;

- Where multiple Holter recordings per patient were available, the highest Lown grade within the study period was used for analysis.
- For patients with clinical arrhythmia or sudden death Holter data obtained prior to the occurrence of primary events were used.

Table 5.
Electrophysiological Data (n=91): Inducible sustained monomorphic VT.

	VT (n=32)	No-VT (n=59)	P *
Age at repair, yrs	8.1 ± 6.6	6.0 ± 6.5	0.154
FU from repair, yrs	20 ± 7.7	15.9 ± 7.5	0.016
VT documented†	20	2	<0.001
AF documented	1	6	0.414
QRS duration, ms	183 ± 22	149 ± 26	<0.001
QRS ≥180 ms	19	5	<0.001
QT dispersion, ms	96 ± 32	58 ± 30	<0.001
Holter, mod. Lown ≥II	16	24	0.244
RVSP (Echo), mmHg	45 ± 18	39 ± 6	0.256
RVOTO (Echo), mmHg	13 ± 13	10 ± 13	0.319
PR moderate (Echo)	27	34	0.012
RV/LV pressure (CC)	0.41 ± 0.15	0.35 ± 0.12	0.069
PS, peripheral (CC)	6	1	0.001

VT= inducible sustained monomorphic ventricular tachycardia; * = by student's t test or chi square test when appropriate; † = with surface ECG at the time of clinical arrhythmia; AF= atrial flutter/fibrillation; Holter, mod. Lown ≥ II= Grade II or greater ventricular arrhythmia on Holter according to the modified Lown Criteria; RVSP= right ventricular systolic pressure; RVOTO= right ventricular outflow tract obstruction; PR= pulmonary regurgitation; RV/LV= right ventricular to left ventricular; PS= pulmonary stenosis cus was located in the area of the infundibulum in 62.5%, at the apex in 12.5%, or both in the remainder. Of the 22 patients with previously documented clinical VT, ventricular stimulation failed to induce sustained monomorphic VT in two patients only (40 and 53 years of age).

Re-Interventions 1985–1995 (Table 6)

Fifty-six patients (7.1%) underwent one or more re-interventions at a mean of 19.8 ± 8.1 (median 18, range 3–32) years from repair. Their age at initial tetralogy of Fallot repair (mean 9.6 ± 8, median 7, range 0.1–45 years) was not different form the rest of the cohort ($p = 0.183$). Surgery was performed in 49, whereas 7 underwent a transcatheter intervention. Five patients underwent multiple interventions (2 in four and 3 in one). One patient died in the early post-operative period, giving a surgical mortality for re-operation of 2%. Clinical arrhythmia preceded re-intervention in 20 patients. Thirteen of them presented with one or more episodes of sustained VT (near-miss sudden death, requiring out of hospital resuscitation in 10) 1 to 12 months prior to re-intervention; the remaining 7 patients presented with atrial flutter/fibrillation 3 months to 3 years prior to intervention.

Follow-up of Patients with Clinical Arrhythmia

Of the 62 patients presenting with clinical arrhythmia during the study period, three patients died from right heart failure, and one from

Table 6. Re-Interventions (1985–1995).			
	Surgical n=49	Catheter n=7	P
Age at repair, years	10.2 ± 8.4	5.8 ± 1.9	0.174
FU from repair, years	19.5 ± 7.6	21.7 ± 11.7	0.501
Procedure			
VSD closure (I)	1	–	
RVOTO enlargement (II)	5 (AF in 1)	–	
PV replacement (III)	21 (VT in 7)	na	
I & II	4 (AF in 2)	–	
II & III	12 (VT in 2, AF in 1) *	na	
I & III	6 (VT in 2, AF in 3)	na	
Balloon dilation of PAs	–	4	
Stenting of PAs	–	3 (VT in 2)	
Ablation †	4 (VT in 3, AF in 1)	2 (VT in 2)	

() = type of clinical arrhythmia preceding the intervention; FU= follow up; VSD= ventricular septal defect; RVOT= right ventricular outflow tract; AF= sustained atrial flutter/fibrillation; PV= pulmonary valve; VT= sustained ventricular tachycardia; * = post-operative death; na= not applicable; PAs= pulmonary arteries; † = not mutually exclusive of other procedures sudden death. None of these four patients underwent re-operations or transcatheter therapy. The patient who died suddenly presented 3 years earlier with atrial flutter, and then syncope (due to VT). Twenty of the remaining patients underwent one or more surgical and/or transcatheter procedures (Table 6); one of them died post-operatively, whereas five had a concomitant ablation for VT and one for atrial flutter. Six patients with VT had an implantable cardioverter-defibrillator as their primary management, without concomitant surgery. The remaining 32 patients were managed medically. At a mean of 3.4 ± 3.4 (median 2, range 0.1 to 9) years of follow-up from presentation with clinical arrhythmia, 57 patients were alive (51 in NYHA functional class I-II and 5 in class III), with overall freedom from arrhythmia recurrence by 1995 of 54%.

Of note, no patient from the 56 who underwent re-intervention, suffered subsequent sudden cardiac death.

Predictors of Clinical Arrhythmia and Sudden Death (Table 7)

By primary analysis, a QRS ≥ 180 msec was predictive of VT and sudden death, whereas age at repair was predictive of sudden death and atrial flutter/fibrillation. Furthermore, a Waterston or Potts anastomosis and the need for reoperation prior to 1985 were predictors of atrial flutter/fibrillation.

Secondary analysis utilizing available longitudinal electrocardiographic and echocardiographic data showed QRS change during the study period to be an additional predictor of VT and sudden death, transannular patch repair for sudden death, and cardiothoracic ratio or moderate to severe tricuspid regurgitation predictors of atrial flutter/fibrillation.

Discussion

This study provides new insights into the pathogenesis and risk stratification for clinical arrhythmia and sudden death, the two major late complications after repair of tetralogy of Fallot. Sustained VT and sudden cardiac death were uncommon, with pulmonary regurgitation being the predominant underlying hemodynamic lesion for both.

Sustained Ventricular Tachycardia

Previous studies have emphasized the relation between impaired post-operative hemodynamics and clinical arrhythmia. An association between RV hypertension and ventricular arrhythmia first noted in 1979[27] was subsequently reported in other series.[28,29] Our study, however, like other more recent studies,[30,31] has failed to show such a relationship, there being no difference in RV systolic pressure between VT and the remaining

Table 7.
Predictors of Ventricular Tachycardia, Sudden Death and Atrial Flutter/Fibrillation After Repair of Tetralogy of Fallot.

Variable	VT (Risk ratio, 95% CI)	P	SD	P	AF	P
Multivariate analysis						
Primary						
Age at repair, years	—		1.07 (1.05–1.10)	<0.0001	1.07 (1.06–1.12)	<0.0001
Waterston or Potts shunt	1.10 (0.32–3.78)		—		9.78 (3.08–31.07)	0.0001
Reintervention prior to 1985	—		—		3.46 (1.49–8.03)	0.004
QRS ≥ 180msec	41.9 (14.7–119.4)	<0.0001	2.29 (1.05–5.02)	0.038	3.39 (1.54–7.47)	
Secondary						
Age at repair, years	—		1.08 (1.02–1.15)	0.009	1.07 (1.03–1.10)	0.0001
Transannular patch	0.18 (0.07–0.49)		11.7 (1.33–103.1)	0.027	—	
QRS ≥ 180msec	8.76 (2.36–32.6)	0.0012	1.08 (0.09–13.07)		0.96 (0.22–4.19)	
QRS annual change, msec	1.08 (1.04–1.10)	<0.001	1.05 (1.02–1.09)	<0.001	2.01 (1.19–3.37)	
Cardiothoracic ratio	0.092 (0.004–0.553)		0.94 (0.71–1.25)		1.12 (1.02–1.26)	0.037
Tricuspid regurgitation, ≥ moderate	0.70 (0.21–2.31)		0.014 (0.002–0.082)		4.66 (1.07–20.29)	0.04

groups. Residual stenoses across the RV outflow tract, as demonstrated by echo Doppler gradients, were modest in the VT and all other groups, suggesting that RV outflow tract obstruction in isolation does not lead to clinical arrhythmogenesis in these patients, at least over 2 decades from repair. It is of note that in past reports, RV hypertension in VT groups was also modest, and the relationship between a raised RV outflow gradient and pulmonary regurgitation (increasing the stroke volume across a not-severely-narrowed outflow tract) was not addressed. Furthermore, the level of obstruction was rarely defined.

More recently, the association of ventricular dysrhythmia to residual pulmonary regurgitation has become apparent.[32–34] Marie et al.[35] demonstrated with electrophysiological studies a strong relationship between inducible sustained VT and increased RV end-diastolic volume, presumably reflecting the effects of residual pulmonary regurgitation.[30] In our study, pulmonary regurgitation was the predominant lesion associated with VT. The use of a transannular patch for RV outflow reconstruction,[36] which in turn creates the potential for free pulmonary regurgitation, was also more common in the VT group and nearly missed significance in being an independent predictor of VT. Approximately half of our VT patients had moderate tricuspid regurgitation, presumably the result of RV and tricuspid annular dilation. Furthermore, there was a relation between inducibility of sustained VT and time from repair, suggesting a possible relationship between a residual, progressive hemodynamic problem and electrophysiological outcome. Peripheral pulmonary artery stenosis was also more common in these patients. It is well known both clinically[33] and experimentally[37] that coexisting peripheral pulmonary stenoses increases pulmonary regurgitation and predisposes to RV dilatation. Our study suggests that distal pulmonary arterial obstruction combined with the anatomic potential for pulmonary regurgitation (i.e., transannular patch repair) may predispose and should be addressed, when assessing risk stratification for VT.

Atrial Flutter/Fibrillation

Patients with atrial flutter/fibrillation were operated later compared to arrhythmia-free and VT patients. Previous Waterston or Potts anastomoses were common in this subgroup. A possible explanation may be that left heart volume overload has contributed to late development of atrial arrhythmia. Re-operation rates were also higher in this compared to all other groups, prior to entering the study. This is in accordance with the report by Roos-Hesselink et al from the Thoraxcenter[38] and our own data,[39] suggesting that patients who went on to develop atrial flutter/fibrillation from these older cohorts may have had a sub-optimal result from initial repair. Not surprisingly, tricuspid regurgitation was the predominant hemodynamic lesion in these patients, presumably leading to right atrial dilation[40] and creating the substrate for atrial arrhythmogenesis.[41] Four patients with atrial flutter/fibrillation developed to VT during the study period; one of them suffered sudden cardiac death. Tricuspid regurgitation per se has the potential to increase RV stroke volume, which, combined with pulmonary regurgitation, may lead to further RV dilatation creating the substrate for ventricular arrhythmogenesis.[14,42]

Sudden Death

Patients with sudden death shared late hemodynamic characteristics with the VT group, underscoring their potential overlap. Their age at repair—like the atrial flutter/fibrillation patients—was greater than the remainder, whereas their cardiothoracic ratio was the largest amongst all groups, reflecting again impaired hemodynamics.[8] Electrocardiographic parameters, like QRS duration and QT dispersion, from the sudden death group were also closer to the VT group, suggesting that, at least in some of the sudden death cases, both RV dilation[14] and the substrate for re-entry tachycardia[15,17,43,44] were present. One could argue that most of the patients with sustained VT from our series (presenting with syncope) could have been victims of sudden cardiac death, should they had not received prompt cardiopulmonary resuscitation.

Although both atrial[38] and ventricular arrhythmias[45,46] have long been recognized after repair of tetralogy, their possible relationship to sudden death has remained uncertain. Our study shows an overlap between sustained VT and sudden death groups, both in terms of residual hemodynamic lesions and electrocardiographic markers, with the potential for sustained VT to lead to sudden death. However, there was only one patient with previous documented VT who subsequently died suddenly from this series. Furthermore, overall prognosis for patients presenting with sustained VT was good, provided that residual hemodynamic lesions were addressed. The main difference, between the VT and sudden death groups was age at repair (the latter underwent repair of tetralogy much later), which may have provided a different myocardial or other substrate. This substrate, which could involve the left ventricle, may have determined a different response to and outcome once VT occurred, i.e., early degeneration to ventricular fibrillation and sudden death in those patients who had a very late repair. It should also be noted that none of the patients who died suddenly, had undergone re-operations during the study period, despite impaired hemodynamics. This is in contrast to patients presenting with atrial flutter/fibrillation and/or VT, in whom surgical or transcatheter procedure/s primarily to restore residual hemodynamic lesions were common.

Risk Stratification & Pathogenesis

Widespread use of ambulatory electrocardiographic (Holter) monitoring has greatly increased the detection of abnormal rhythm patterns in these patients. In some centers, when ventricular ectopy exceeded a certain limit (e.g. > 30 ventricular premature beats per hour), otherwise asymptomatic patients have been commenced on prophylactic antiarrhythmic treatment. The wisdom of this approach has been questioned.[47] Even if ventricular ectopy was a reliable marker of patients susceptibility to sustained VT and sudden death, the value of treatment to suppress this marker has never been shown. Indeed, given the findings of the CAST study[48] in adults after myocardial infarction, routine antiarrhythmic therapy in low risk groups may be more harmful than no therapy. Our study provides additional evidence that both frequency and complexity of ventricular ectopy on Holter does not relate to inducibility of VT at electrophysiological studies and has no predictive value for clinical VT and sudden death. Studies that report results of Holter monitoring as endpoints for the incidence of arrhythmia (e.g., after different surgical strategies for repair of tetralogy) must, therefore, be interpreted with caution.

Electrocardiographic markers previously shown to be predictive of sustained VT[14–16] and sudden death[14,17] were validated in our multi-center study and found to retain their relative sensitivity and specificity. Furthermore, this study confirmed the previously reported association between QRS duration and cardiothoracic ratio from chest radiograph.[14,49] A large heart and a prolonged QRS duration are ominous signs, probably interrelated, underscoring the proposed mechano-electric interaction[14,49–52] of residual hemodynamic abnormalities leading to specific electrophysiological sequelae.[42] Marked QT dispersion in the VT and sudden death groups is highly suggestive of a re-entry mechanism for clinical arrhythmogenesis in these patients.[15,44] The focus of VT was at the RV outflow tract in the majority of patients; however, over one-third of patients had the VT focus at the apex or at multiple sites. This suggests a more widespread abnormality of electrical activity,[50] perhaps due to global myocardial "damage" and stretch, rather than a problem confined only to the area of surgical scar. The QRS prolongation[14,51] seen in these patients is only in part due to the acute effect of surgery,[53] whereas the rest develops over a long period of time and relates to RV dilation.[14,39,52] This QRS prolongation with time may be of greater importance to outcome and of particular relevance to contemporary series in whom repair is often performed via the transatrial/transpulmonary approach, as opposed to the ventricular route to repair used for the majority of the patients reported here. Transatrial repair has already been shown to lead to less QRS prolongation immediately after surgery, by limiting the extent of right ventriculotomy and therefore the damage to the right bundle branch. A late and rapid increase in QRS length during the study was observed primarily in patients who developed VT or suffered sudden death. This was in contrast to patients who developed atrial flutter/fibrillation, previously shown[39] to have a marked and early postoperative increase in QRS duration, who during this study had a constant albeit slower rate of QRS prolongation. It may be that, when a certain threshold of RV dilatation and stretch is exceeded, the electrical conditions for re-entry are met and clinical arrhythmogenesis follows. It should be remembered, however, that many potential mechanisms for sudden death exist in this population. Atrial flutter, complete heart block, "vascular catastrophe,"[12] and others may play a role. Therefore no theory or risk stratification can truly be all-embracing.

Limitations

Many patients from this study reflect the outcome of early eras of surgery, performed by different surgeons, with different techniques. It may be that newer surgical strategies will influence outcome.[4,11,34,55] The incidence of right bundle branch block, for example, has been reduced by the transatrial/transpulmonary approach to repair.[34,56,57] The timing and nature of surgery in contemporary series may also affect the mechano-electrical relation reported here. Furthermore, this is a retrospective, uncontrolled study with a potential for selection bias because of the nature of referrals. Nevertheless, it reflects large numbers of such patients currently presenting in adult life.[58] Prospective studies with standardized data collection may uncover additional predictors of such devastating clinical events.

In conclusion, our study has several important clinical implications. The electrophysiological and hemodynamic substrate of sudden death in this cohort of late follow-up patients with repaired tetralogy was close to that of sustained VT. Older age at repair in the sudden death group was their main difference. Pulmonary regurgitation was the main underlying hemodynamic lesion for both. Preservation or restoration of pulmonary valve function[59-61] may thus be important in reducing the risk of sudden death. ECG markers, possibly as a surrogate or directly related, can help select patients at risk. These data cannot support the use of routine Holter monitoring for risk stratification of VT and sudden death after repair of tetralogy of Fallot.

Annexe

Since the study has been concluded,[62] there have been reports showing that pulmonary valve replacement—with or without concomitant cryoablation—impacts on pre-existing arrhythmia[63-65] and modifies the risk for sudden cardiac death in these patients by stabilizing the QRS duration.[65] As discussed by Drs. Saul and Blaufox in Chapter III and Dr. Graham in Chapter IV, restoration of RV outflow competence with timely pulmonary valve implantation has a positive impact on RV function. The latter should also be considered, when stratifying for arrhythmia and sudden cardiac death late after repair of tetralogy.

In our practice at the Royal Brompton Hospital, we employ both absolute QRS duration and recent QRS change in combination with thorough assessment of underlying hemodynamics for our risk stratification for sustained VT and sudden cardiac death for our adults with previous tetralogy repair. Restoration of residual hemodynamic problems is our first therapeutic goal for patients at risk, or those presenting with arrhythmia. Of note, patients with documented atrial flutter/fibrillation may still be at risk of sustained VT. We reserve Holter monitoring and invasive electrophysiologic studies for symptomatic patients investigated for arrhythmia. Internal cardioverter defibrillators (ICDs) are playing an increasing role for secondary prevention of sustained VT and near-miss sudden cardiac death. ICDs are also considered for primary prevention for patients at risk (with QRS > 180 ms, recent change in QRS duration, advanced ventricular dysfunction) without target hemodynamic lesions amenable to re-interventions.

References

1. Lillehei CW, Cohen M, Warden HE, et al. Direct vision intracardiac surgical correction of the tetralogy of Fallot, pentalogy of Fallot, and pulmonary atresia defects: Report of first ten cases. *Ann Surg* 1955;142:418–445.
2. Kirklin JW, DuShane JW, Patrick RT, et al. Intracardiac surgery with the aid of a mechanical pump-oxygenator system (Gibbon type): Report of eight cases. *Mayo Clin Proc* 1955;30:201–206.
3. Murphy JG, Gersh BJ, Mair DD, et al. Long-term outcome in patients undergoing surgical repair of tetralogy of Fallot. *N Engl J Med* 1993;329:593–599.
4. Karl TR, Pornviliwan S, Mee RBB. Tetralogy of Fallot: Favourable outcome of non-neonatal transatrial, transpulmonary repair. *Ann Thorac Surg* 1992;54:903–907.
5. Lillehei CW, Varco RL, Cohen M, et al. The first open heart corrections of tetralogy of Fallot: A 26–31 year follow-up of 106 patients. *Ann Surg* 1986;204:490–502.
6. Katz NM, Blackstone EH, Kirklin JW, et al. Late survival and symptoms after repair of tetralogy of Fallot. *Circulation* 1982;65:403–410.
7. Rosing DR, Borer JS, Kent KM, et al. Long-term hemodynamic and electrocardiographic assessment following operative repair of tetralogy of Fallot. *Circulation* 1978;58(suppl I):I-209-I-217.
8. Garson A, McNamara DG. Sudden death in a paediatric cardiology population: Relationship to prior arrhythmias. *J Am Coll Cardiol* 1988;5:134B-137B.
9. Deanfield JE, McKenna WJ, Presbitero P, et al. Ventricular arrhythmia in unrepaired and repaired tetralogy of Fallot. Relation to age, timing of repair, and heamodynamic status. *Br Heart J* 1984;52:77–81.
10. Kavey RE, Thomas D, Byrum CJ, et al. Ventricular arrhythmias and biventricular dysfunction after repair of tetralogy of Fallot. *J Am Coll Cardiol* 1984;4:126–131.
11. Castaneda AR, Freed MD, Williams RG, et al. Repair of tetralogy of Fallot in infancy: Early and late results. *J Thorac Cardiovasc Surg* 1977;74:372–381.
12. Bricker JT. Sudden death and tetralogy of Fallot: Risks, markers, and causes. *Circulation* 1995;92:158–159.
13. Garson A, Randall DG, Gillette PC, et al. Prevention of sudden death after repair of tetralogy of Fallot: Treatment of ventricular arrhythmias. *J Am Coll Cardiol* 1985;6:221–227.

14. Gatzoulis MA, Till JA, Somerville J, et al. Mechano-electrical interaction in tetralogy of Fallot: QRS prolongation relates to right ventricular size and predicts malignant ventricular arrhythmias and sudden death. *Circulation* 1995;92:231–237.
15. Gatzoulis MA, Till JA, Redington AN. Depolarisation-repolarisation inhomogeneity after repair of tetralogy of Fallot: The substrate for malignant ventricular tachycardia? *Circulation* 1997;95:401–404.
16. Balaji S, Lau YR, Case CL, et al. QRS prolongation is associated with inducible ventricular tachycardia after repair of tetralogy of Fallot. *Am J Cardiol* 1997; 80:160–163.
17. Berul CI, Hill SL, Geggel RL, et al. Electrocardiographic markers of late sudden death risk in postoperative tetralogy of Fallot children. *J Cardiovasc Electrophysiol* 1997;8:1349–1356.
18. Kugler JD. Predicting sudden death in patients who have undergone tetralogy of Fallot repair: Is it really as simple as measuring ECG intervals? *J Cardiovasc Electrophysiol* 1998;9:103–106.
19. Day CP, McComb JM, Campbell RWF. QT dispersion: An indication of arrhythmia in risk patients with long QT intervals. *Br Heart J* 1990;63:342–344.
20. Pye M, Quinn AC, Cobbe SM. QT interval dispersion: A non-invasive marker of susceptibility to arrhythmia in patients with sustained ventricular arrhythmias? *Br Heart J* 1994;71:511–514.
21. Barr CS, Naas A, Freeman M, et al. QT dispersion and sudden unexpected death in chronic heart failure. *Lancet* 1994;343:327–329.
22. Ryan M, Lown B, Horn H. Comparison of ventricular ectopic activity during the 24 hour monitoring and exercise testing in patients with coronary heart disease. *N Engl J Med* 1975;292:224–229.
23. Deanfield JE, McKenna WJ, Hallidie-Smith KA. Detection of late arrhythmia and conduction disturbance after correction of tetralogy of Fallot. *Br Heart J* 1980;44:248–253.
24. Wellens HJJ, Brugada P, Stevenson WG. Programmed electrical stimulation of the heart in patients with life-threatening ventricular arrhythmias: What is the significance of induced arrhythmias and what is the correct stimulation protocol? *Circulation* 1985;72:1–7.
25. Cox DR. Regression models and life tables. *J Royal Stat Soc (B)* 1972;34:187–220.
26. Gillette PC, Yeoman MA, Mullins CE, et al. Sudden death after repair of tetralogy of Fallot: Electrocardiographic and electrophysiologic abnormalities. *Circulation* 1977;56:566–571.
27. Garson A, Nihill MR, McNamara DG, et al. Status of the adult and adolescent after repair of tetralogy of Fallot. *Circulation* 1979;59:1232–1240.
28. Katz NM, Blackstone EH, Kirklin JW, et al. Late survival and symptoms after repair of tetralogy of Fallot. *Circulation* 1982;65:403–410.
29. Kobayashi J, Hirose H, Nakano S, et al. Ambulatory electrocardiographic study of the frequency and cause of ventricular arrhythmia after correction of tetralogy of Fallot. *Am J Cardiol* 1984;54:1310–1313.
30. Zahka KG, Horneffer PJ, Rowe SA, et al. Long-term valvular function after total repair of tetralogy of Fallot: Relation to ventricular arrhythmias. *Circulation* 1988;78(suppl III):III-14-III-19.
31. Harrison DA, Harris L, Siu SC, et al. Sustained ventricular tachycardia in adult patients late after repair of tetralogy of Fallot. *J Am Coll Cardiol* 1997; 30:1368–1373.
32. Bove EL, Byrum CJ, Thomas FD, et al. The influence of pulmonary insufficiency on ventricular function following repair of tetralogy of Fallot. *J Thorac Cardiovasc Surg* 1983;85:691–696.

33. Ilbawi MN, Idriss FS, DeLeon SY, et al. Factors that exaggerate the deleterious effects of pulmonary insufficiency on the right ventricle after tetralogy repair. *J Thorac Cardiovasc Surg* 1987;93:36–44.
34. Dietl CA, Cazzaniga ME, Dubner SJ, et al. Life-threatening arrhythmias and RV dysfunction after surgical repair of tetralogy of Fallot: Comparison between transventricular and transatrial approaches. *Circulation* 1994;90(part 2):II-7–II-12.
35. Marie PY, Marcon F, Brunotte F, et al. Right ventricular overload and induced sustained ventricular tachycardia in operatively "repaired" tetralogy of Fallot. *Am J Cardiol* 1992;69:785–789.
36. Kirklin JK, Kirklin JW, Blackstone EH, et al. Effect of transannular patching on outcome after repair of tetralogy of Fallot. *Ann Thorac Surg* 1989;48:783–791.
37. Chaturvedi RR, Kilner P, White P, et al. Increased airway pressure and simulated branch pulmonary stenosis increase pulmonary regurgitation after repair of tetralogy of Fallot: Real-time analysis using conductance catheter technique. *Circulation* 1997;95:643–649.
38. Roos-Hesselink J, Perlroth MG, McGhie J, et al. Atrial arrhythmias in adults after repair of tetralogy of Fallot: Correlations with clinical, exercise, and echocardiographic findings. *Circulation* 1995;91:2214–2219.
39. Till JA, Gatzoulis MA, Deanfield JE, et al. Evolution of QRS prolongation following repair of tetralogy of Fallot: Implications for symptomatic arrhythmia and sudden death. *Circulation* 1995;92(suppl):I-707.
40. Satoh T, Zipes DP. Unequal atrial stretch increase dispersion of refractoriness conducive to developing atrial fibrillation. *J Cardiovasc Electrophysiol* 1996;7:833–842.
41. Morillo CA, Klein GJ, Jones DL, et al. Chronic rapid atrial pacing: Structural, functional and electrophysiological characteristics of a new model of sustained atrial fibrillation. *Circulation* 1995;91:1588–1595.
42. Dean JW, Lab MJ. Arrhythmia in heart failure: Role of mechanically induced changes in electrophysiology. *Lancet* 1989;1:1309–1311.
43. Lab M. Transient depolarisations and action potential alterations following mechanical changes in isolated myocardium. *Cardiovasc Res* 1980;14:624–637.
44. Downar E, Harris L, Kimber S, et al. Ventricular tachycardia after surgical repair of tetralogy of Fallot: Results of intraoperative mapping studies. *J Am Coll Cardiol* 1992;20:648–655.
45. Garson A, Porter CJ, Gillette PC, et al. Induction of ventricular tachycardia during electrophysiologic study after repair of tetralogy of Fallot. *J Am Coll Cardiol* 1983;1:1493–1502.
46. Kugler JD, Pinsky WW, Cheatham JP, et al. Sustained ventricular tachycardia after repair of Fallot: New electrophysiologic findings. *Am J Cardiol* 1983;51:1137–1143.
47. Cullen S, Celermajer DS, Franklin RCG, et al. Prognostic significance of ventricular arrhythmia after repair of tetralogy of Fallot: A 12-year prospective study. *J Am Coll Cardiol* 1994;23:1151–1155.
48. The cardiac arrhythmia suppression study (CAST) investigators. Preliminary report: Effect of encainide on mortality in a randomized trial of arrhythmia suppression after myocardial infarction. *N Engl J Med* 1989;321:406–412.
49. Abd El Rahman MY, Abdul-Khaliq H, Vogel M, et al. Relation between right ventricular enlargement, QRS duration, and right ventricular function in patients with tetralogy of Fallot and pulmonary regurgitation after surgical repair. *Heart* 2000;84:416–420.
50. Deanfield J, McKenna W, Rowland E. Local abnormalities of right ventricular depolarisation after repair of tetralogy of Fallot: A basis for ventricular arrhythmia. *Am J Cardiol* 1985;55:522–525.

51. Davignon A, Rautaharju P, Boiselle E, et al. Normal ECG standards for infants and children. *Pediatr Cardiol* 1979/80;1:123–131.
52. d'Udekem Y, Ovaert C, Grandjean F, et al. Tetralogy of fallot: Transannular and right ventricular patching equally affect late functional status. *Circulation* 2000;102[suppl III]:III-116–III-122.
53. Norgard G, Gatzoulis MA, Moraes F, et al. The relationship between type of outflow tract repair and postoperative right ventricular diastolic physiology in tetralogy of Fallot: Implications for long-term outcome *Circulation* 1996;94:3276–3281.
54. Graham TP, Cordell D, Atwood GF, et al. Right ventricular volume characteristics before and after palliative and reparative operation in tetralogy of Fallot. *Circulation* 1976;54:417–423.
55. Kawashima Y, Kitamura S, Nakano S, et al. Corrective surgery for tetralogy of Fallot without or with minimal right ventriculotomy and with repair of the pulmonary valve. *Circulation* 1981;64(suppl 2):147–153.
56. Atallah-Yunes NH, Kavey RW, Bove EL, et al. Postoperative assessment of modified surgical approach to repair of tetralogy of Fallot: Long-term follow-up. *Circulation* 1996;94:II-22-II-26.
57. Munkhammar P, Cullen S, Jogi P, et al. Early age at repair prevents restrictive right ventricular physiology after surgery for tetralogy of Fallot: Diastolic RV function after TOF repair in infancy. *J Am Coll Cardiol* 1998;32:1083–1087.
58. Rosenthal A. Adults with tetralogy of Fallot: Repaired, yes: Cured, no. *N Engl J Med* 1993;329:655–656.
59. Bove EL, Kavey RW, Byrum CJ, et al. Improved right ventricular function following late pulmonary valve replacement for residual pulmonary insufficiency or stenosis. *J Thorac Cardiovasc Surg* 1985;90:50–55.
60. Warner KG, Anderson JE, Fulton DR, et al. Restoration of the pulmonary valve reduces right ventricular volume overload after previous repair of tetralogy of Fallot. *Circulation* 1993;88[part 2]:189–197.
61. Yemets IM, Williams WG, Webb GD, et al. Pulmonary valve replacement late after repair of tetralogy of Fallot. *Ann Thorac Surg* 1997;64:526–530.
62. Gatzoulis MA, Balaji S, Webber SA, et al. Risk factors for arrhythmia and sudden death in repaired tetralogy of Fallot: A multi-centre study. *The Lancet* 2000; 356:975–981.
63. Oechslin EN, Harrison DA, Harris L, et al. Reoperation in adults with repair of Tetralogy of Fallot: Indications and outcomes. *J Thorac Cardiovasc Surg* 1999;118:245–251.
64. Discigil B, Dearani JA, Puga FJ, et al. Late pulmonary valve replacement after repair of tetralogy of Fallot. *J Thorac Cardiovasc Surg* 2001;121:344–351.
65. Therrien J, Siu SC, Harris L, et al. Impact of pulmonary valve replacement on arrhythmia propensity late after repair of tetralogy of Fallot. *Circulation* 2001;104 (in press).

Chapter II

Catheter Interventions in Tetralogy of Fallot

Peter McLaughlin

Introduction

Over the past two decades a wide variety of catheter interventional techniques have been developed. Many of these techniques have been effective in the management of patients with tetralogy of Fallot, both before and after intracardiac repair. By nature, most of these catheter interventions are performed in the cardiac catheterization lab by the interventionalist. However, the congenital cardiac surgeon in the cardiac operating room, as an adjunct to direct suture repair, may use some of these techniques effectively. The arsenal of the interventionist and surgeon includes balloon-only angioplasty, balloon angioplasty with stenting, and use of coils, umbrellas, and other occlusive devices. This chapter will review these techniques and the outcomes that may be anticipated.

Branch Pulmonary Artery Stenosis

Balloon angioplasty alone and with stenting has become the mainstay of treatment for branch pulmonary stenosis. In 1983 Lock et al.[1] described balloon dilation angioplasty of branch pulmonary artery stenosis in a series of seven patients. Further small series of balloon dilation angioplasty were published from 1984 to 1986.[2,3] Complications in these early series included vessel perforation, unilateral pulmonary edema, and late aneurysm formation. In 1990, the results of 182 procedures in branch pulmonary stenosis were published from the Valvuloplasty and Angioplasty for Congenital Anomalies (VACA) Registry.[4] Complications included five deaths in 156 patients with vessel perforation in two; low cardiac output, paradoxical embolism, and cardiac arrest in three. Three patients had nonfatal pulmonary hemorrhage. In 1992, Hosking, Benson and co-workers

From Gatzoulis MA, Murphy DJ (eds): *The Adult with Tetralogy of Fallot: The ISACCD Monograph Series* ©Futura Publishing Co., Inc, Armonk, NY, 2001.

from the Hospital for Sick Children in Toronto reported the results of 110 balloon angioplasty procedures for branch stenosis in 72 patients.[5] They reported a 53% success rate with a 5% complication rate. Subsequent experience with high-pressure balloons showed improved results with success up to 81%.[6]

The use of balloon expandable stainless steel stents in patients with congenital heart disease was first reported by O'Laughlin et al. in 1991,[7] with a larger series of 121 stents in 85 patients in 1993 from the same group.[8] Benson and co-workers reported the results of 55 stents in 42 patients with branch pulmonary artery stenosis in 1995.[9] Stenting of pulmonary arteries has been an important advance in treatment of this problem, and allows effective and safer dilation with control of the intimal tear. The complications of stenting in the pulmonary circulation have been reported to include migration of the stent beyond the intended target, thrombosis within the stent and distal to the stent, occasional side-branch occlusion, retroperitoneal hemorrhage, and rarely, death from pulmonary hemorrhage or unilateral pulmonary edema.[9–11] The occurrence of migration has been related to patient selection and experience, and is uncommon in later series. In this situation the stent is usually deployed in a benign position and the target is stented again. There are conflicting reports of the frequency of restenosis after stenting pulmonary arteries; however, Benson's report indicated that 15 of 55 stents required redilation, suggesting the need for on-going follow-up of these patients.

Figure 1 illustrates the use of balloon angioplasty with stenting in a 26-year-old man with tetralogy of Fallot who had undergone intracardiac repair at age 15. The gradient across the right pulmonary stenosis was 50 mmHg before stenting, and was reduced to no gradient after stenting.

Conduit Stenosis

Stenting of right ventricular to pulmonary artery conduits after intracardiac repair of tetralogy is somewhat more problematic than branch pulmonary stenosis, but can be effective in selected patients where deferral of surgical replacement is the preferred management. Initial reports from 1990 to 1993 indicated the feasibility of the procedure and the potential to reduce the gradient across the conduit.[8,12,13] Benson and co-workers reported their experience from 1990 to 1997 with stent implantation in forty-three obstructed conduits. The median age at procedure was 6 years, and the median interval between conduit insertion and stent implantation was 2.4 years. Mean systolic right ventricular pressures decreased from 71 ± 18 mmHg to 48 ± 15 mmHg, and mean gradients decreased from 48 ± 19 mmHg to 19 ± 13 mmHg after stent placement. Fifteen patients underwent a second transcatheter intervention, either dilation or additional stenting, and two patients underwent a third catheter

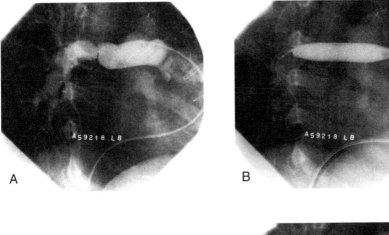

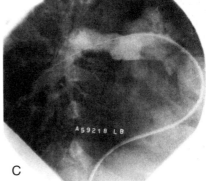

Figure 1. Figure 1A shows the predilation angiogram of the right pulmonary artery with a gradient of 50 mmHg. Figure 1B shows the balloon angioplasty and stenting of the stenosis. Figure 1C shows the post dilation result with no residual stenosis.

intervention. Freedom from surgical re-intervention was 86% at 1 year, 72% at 2 years, and 47% at 4 years. Complications appear to be rare with this treatment. Limitations of this approach include the large sheaths required to introduce the stents, sub-optimal results from further transcatheter re-interventions in the conduit, and resultant free pulmonary insufficiency after stent implantation. The pulmonary regurgitation is aggravated by more distal obstruction and underlines the importance of assessing the pulmonary flow run-off and treating distal branch stenosis if present. Stenting of conduit stenosis is less effective in some situations, including the setting of long-standing stenosis, absence of discrete stenosis, and small conduits. There is a distinct learning curve, which will affect outcome. The advantages of conduit stenting include its safety, moderate effectiveness in many patients, the benefits of deferring conduit replacement for a variable time, and the fact that conduit stenting does not compromise the surgical procedure when it is eventually performed.

To summarize, stenting of obstructed conduits may delay the need for

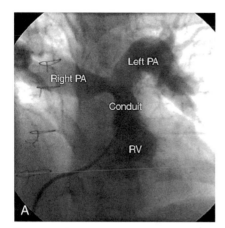
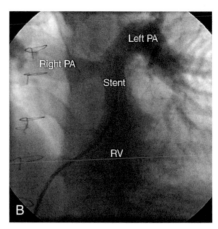

Figure 2. Figure 2A shows an angiogram of the right ventricular to pulmonary artery conduit with narrowing at the distal end of the conduit. The prestent gradient was 30 mmHg by catheter pull-back. Figure 2B shows the conduit after implantation of the stent. The post-stent gradient was reduced to 12 mmHg.

surgical replacement in selected patients, and so may be helpful in decreasing the number of cardiac operations in some patients. The procedure must be viewed as a palliative procedure, and is not a replacement for eventual surgical treatment. Figure 2 illustrates the case of a 23-year-old man with type 1 truncus arteriosus at birth who had a right ventricular to pulmonary artery conduit implanted at age 1, replacement of the conduit at age 6, and replacement of the second conduit at age 14. Between age 20 and 23 there was a progressive increase in the conduit gradient to a peak doppler gradient of 70 mmHg, with shortness of breath on exertion. Diagnostic heart catheterization showed right ventricular pressures of 64/13 mmHg, and pulmonary artery pressures of 34/16/21 mmHg. Angiography showed calcification and narrowing at the site of the valve, with additional narrowing at the origin of the right pulmonary artery (Figure 2a). The decision was made to stent the conduit as a strategy to defer replacement for the time being. Post stenting (Figure 2b) the gradient was reduced to 12 mmHg, and the right ventricular systolic pressure was 44 mmHg.

Residual Shunts

Unwanted residual shunts after repair of tetralogy are usually best managed by catheter intervention. These shunts may include Blalock-Taussig shunts that have recanalized, or could not be taken down at reparative surgery. There are different approaches to closing these shunts, including use of umbrella devices or plugs, coils, or coils combined with spider devices to prevent embolization.

Figure 3 illustrates the case of a 36-year-old man who was born with tetralogy of Fallot. He had a left Blalock-Taussig shunt at age 2 years and an intra-cardiac repair at age 10 years with take-down of the shunt using triple ligation. Recanalization of the shunt was noted at age eleven, and he was observed. By adulthood heart size was noted to be increasing, and an initial attempt was made to insert a coil into the shunt at his home hospital. This coil embolized to this left lung. He was referred to the University of Toronto Congenital Cardiac Centre for surgical closure, and the decision was made to approach the shunt with catheter intervention. Shunt angiogram showed a diameter of 4–6 mm (Figure 3a). A 13-mm Amplatz spider was positioned at the distal end of the shunt (Figures 3b, 3c). Two coils

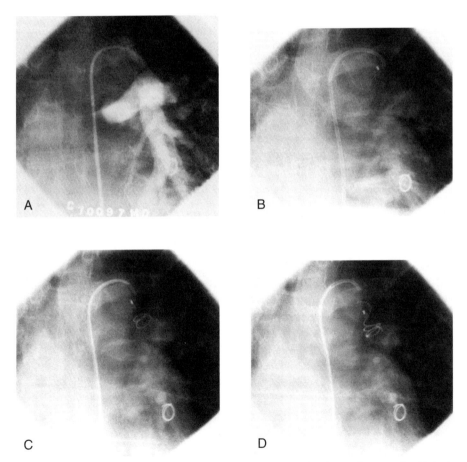

Figure 3. A 36-year-old man with residual Blalock-Taussig shunt after repair of tetralogy (3A). An Amplatz spider was positioned in the distal end of the shunt (3B), and followed by two 8-mm coils (3C,3D) *continued*

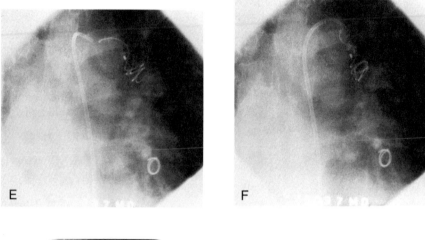

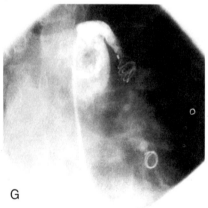

Figure 3. *Continued* Two 5-mm coils (3E,3F). The final angiogram shows complete closure (3G).

of 8-mm diameter were wrapped around the spider, followed by two 5-mm coils proximal to the spider (Figures 3d, 3e). This resulted in immediate and complete closure of the shunt (Figure 3f, 3g).

Aorto-Pulmonary Arteries

Aorto-pulmonary arteries that require closure either for excessive volume overload of the left ventricle, or as a preoperative strategy, can often be effectively managed in the catheter lab. Figure 4 illustrates the case of a 21-year-old man who had surgical closure of a patent ductus arteriosus at age 2 days. Persistent continuous murmurs were found after surgery. By age 8 years, his parents noted poor performance at school, and the heart size was enlarging on chest x-ray. An aorto-pulmonary artery to the right lung was found on angiography and embolized with coils. The patient re-

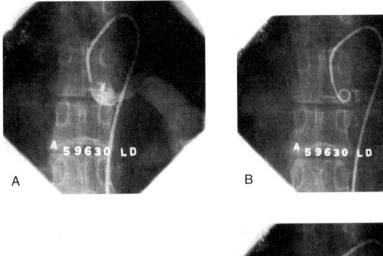

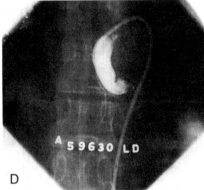

Figure 4. 21-year-old man with recurrent large aorto-pulmonary arteries to the right and left lung. Figure 4A shows the large aorto-pulmonary to the left lung. Coils are inserted in Figure 4B, and the final angiogram showing complete closure is illustrated in Figure 4C.

mained asymptomatic through adolescence. By age 18, functional capacity was reduced, with mild dyspnea on exertion. He had a cough productive of sputum and had had one episode of hemoptysis. Continuous murmurs were again heard, but over the left precordium and back. Diagnostic heart catheterization demonstrated large aorto-pulmonary arteries to both the right and left lung. Figures 4a to 4c show the aorto-pulmonary artery to the left lung before embolization, insertion of the coils, and the final angiogram after closure.

Combined Catheter-Surgical Strategies

There are some instances where the patient may benefit from a combined catheter intervention-surgical strategy. Kreutzer, Lock and co-workers reported on ten patients with tetralogy in 1996. Balloon dilation of the pulmonary valve and arteries, along with coil embolization of aorto-pulmonary collaterals was carried out prior to surgery. Growth of pulmonary arteries was documented, and the elimination of aorto-pulmonary arteries facilitated later surgical repair.[14] Pagani and co-workers have also reported combined strategies for optimum treatment, and a treatment algorithm for patients with tetralogy of Fallot and pulmonary trunk atresia and diminutive pulmonary arteries.[15]

In our own center, our congenital cardiovascular surgeons frequently implant stents in the pulmonary arteries during surgical repair to improve vessel diameter. Thus, catheter interventions, while usually done in the cardiac cath lab by interventional cardiologists, can be an equally important tool in the surgical armamentarium.

References

1. Lock JE, Castaneda-Zuniga WR, Fuhrman BP, et al. Balloon dilation angioplasty of hypoplastic and stenotic pulmonary arteries. *Circulation* 1983;67:962–967.
2. Rocchini AP, Kveselis D, Dick M, et al. Use of balloon angioplasty to treat peripheral pulmonary stenosis. *Am J Cardiol* 1984;54:1069–1073.
3. Bass JL. Percutaneous balloon dilation angioplasty of pulmonary artery branch stenosis. *Cardiovasc Intervent Radiol* 1986;9:299–302.
4. Kan JS, Marvin Jr WJ, Bass JL, et al. Balloon angioplasty-branch pulmonary artery stenosis: Results from the Valvuloplasty and Angioplasty of Congenital Anomalies Registry. *Am J Cardiol* 1990;65:798–801.
5. Hosking MC, Thomaidis C, Hamilton R, et al. Clinical impact of balloon angioplasty for branch pulmonary arterial stenosis. *Am J Cardiol* 1992;69:1467–1470.
6. Gentles TL, Lock JE, Perry SB. High pressure balloon angioplasty for branch pulmonary artery stenosis: Early experience. *JACC* 1993;22:867–872.
7. O'Laughlin MP, Perry SB, Lock JE, et al. Use of endovascular stents in congenital heart disease. *Circulation* 1991;83:1923–1939.
8. O'Laughlin MR, Slack MC, Grifka RG, et al. Implantation and intermediate-term follow-up of stents in congenital heart disease. *Circulation* 1993;88:605–614.
9. Fogelman R, Nykanen D, Smallhorn JF, et al. Endovascular stents in the pulmonary circulation. *Circulation* 1995;92:881–885.
10. O'Laughlin MP. Catheterization treatment of stenosis and hypoplasia of pulmonary arteries. *Pediatric Cardiol* 1998;19:48–56.
11. Shaffer KM, Mullins CI, Grifka RG, et al. Intravascular stents in congenital heart disease: Short- and long-term results from a large, single-center experience. *JACC* 1998; 31: 661–667.
12. Almagor Y, Prevosti LG, Bartorelli AL, et al. Balloon expandable stent implantation in stenotic right heart valved conduits. *JACC* 990;16:1310–1314.
13. Hosking MCK, Benson LN, Nakanishi T, et al. Intravascular stent prosthesis for right ventricular outflow obstruction. *JACC* 992;20:373–380.
14. Kreutzer J, Perry SB, Jonas RA, et al. Tetralogy of Fallot with diminutive pulmonary arteries: Preoperative pulmonary valve dilation and transcatheter rehabilitation of pulmonary arteries. *JACC* 1996;27:1741–1747.
15. Pagani FD, Cheatham JP, Beekman III RH, et al. The management of tetralogy of Fallot with pulmonary atresia and diminutive pulmonary arteries. *J Thorac Cardiovasc Surg* 1995;110:1521–1532.

Chapter III

Cardiopulmonary Exercise Performance in Tetralogy of Fallot

Derize Boshoff, Tony Reybrouck, Marc Gewillig

Introduction

Most patients have an excellent functional result after surgical repair of tetralogy of Fallot, with dramatic improvement of their clinical status and quality of life.[1-3] Measurement of physical activity is usually performed as routine part of the patient's cardiac evaluation; exercise testing of patients with congenital heart disease in general and tetralogy in particular, has had much less impact on clinical care until recently than that of adults with coronary heart disease. Exercise testing unmasks the presence and severity of residual cardiovascular abnormalities, and has contributed significantly to the understanding of the natural history and pathophysiology of surgically corrected tetralogy, thus optimizing management.[4]

In this chapter we will concentrate on the following aspects regarding cardiopulmonary exercise performance in patients with repaired tetralogy: why objective exercise testing is necessary, measurement of work performance, heart rate response, importance of residual right ventricular (RV) outflow obstruction and pulmonary regurgitation, the role of biventricular function, arrhythmias and exercise, lung function and ventilatory response to exercise, and the role of physical training in improving exercise performance.

Subjective Estimates of Exercise Performance

Clinicians often rely on questionnaires and patient history for the assessment of physical activity, but it has been shown that self-reports are

From Gatzoulis MA, Murphy DJ (eds): *The Adult with Tetralogy of Fallot: The ISACCD Monograph Series* ©Futura Publishing Co., Inc, Armonk, NY, 2001.

inherently biased. Subjects often underestimate their participation in sedentary activity and grossly overestimate their participation in aerobic activity.[5] Comparisons between clinical estimates of exercise capacity and measured values, showed weak correlations in a group of adult patients complaining mostly of chest pain and dyspnea. Clinical estimates tended to be lower than measured values in the majority of cases.[6] Rogers et al.[7] compared subjective assessments of activity level (self-reporting and use of standardized questionnaires) to objective measurement of exercise capacity, obtained from respiratory gas exchange measurements during submaximal exercise testing (ventilatory threshold method) in 69 children after total correction of tetralogy. The outcome of surgery was considered to be very good, based on clinical findings. All patients were symptom-free, participated in daily physical activities, and were attending school normally, but none were engaged in competitive sports or heavy physical activities. The majority of patients in this study (69%) would have been misclassified based on subjective estimates of exercise capacity. As a group, parents overestimated their child's exercise capacity, as could have been expected. A high level of physical activity in daily life is often confused with a high level of exercise performance. Important variables to consider are duration of exercise, frequency of movement, and intensity of physical activity. Each of these variables alone, or in combination, results in different caloric expenditure and physiologic outcomes.[8] Exercise testing should therefore be regarded as an integral part of the long-term evaluation of patients with tetralogy of Fallot after surgical correction, because it provides quantitative, numerical, reproducible information about the patient's ability to perform physical work.[4]

Objective Assessment of Work Performance

Exercise capacity following complete repair of tetralogy has been the object of many studies.[4,9] There has been uniform agreement that, as a group, patients with repaired tetralogy have mild to moderate reduction in aerobic capacity, although individual variations are large.[10–18] The cause of this impaired aerobic capacity remains elusive.[9] Residual RV outflow obstruction, pulmonary regurgitation, RV systolic and diastolic dysfunction, chronotropic impairment, pulmonary artery hypoplasia, and physical deconditioning have all been implicated as possible etiologies for aerobic impairment.

In reviewing the data on exercise studies in tetralogy, one is struck by the wide range of different approaches and the lack of uniform standards for exercise testing in patients with congenital heart disease.[4] Determination of maximal oxygen uptake (VO_{2max}) is dependent on motivation of both the patient and the investigator.

Work capacity is best evaluated by maximal exercise.[4] The data should be expressed as percentage of predicted known standards or simultaneously studied normal controls and/or in terms of the VO_{2max}, conventionally expressed in mL/min/kg body weight.[4]

Submaximal exercise levels are more relevant to daily life activities. For submaximal exercise tests the determination of VO_2 at the ventilatory anaerobic threshold (VAT) should be used, since VO_2 at VAT defines the limits of endurance performance and correlates well with VO_{2max}.[4,19-22] Normal standards for VAT in healthy children and adolescents have been reported.[23] Calculation of the VAT can be influenced by several factors that increase the variance of the result, including differences in the exercise protocol, the method used for threshold determination, and interobserver differences.[24-26] During submaximal exercise testing, the adequacy of the O_2 transport system can be more specifically evaluated by assessment of the steepness of the slope of oxygen uptake versus exercise intensity (SVO_2), also expressed in mL O_2/min/kg.[27,28] A typical example of the slope of the VO_2 versus exercise intensity is shown in Figure 1.

When objectively evaluated, work capacity remains markedly impaired after shunt palliation.[29,30] Work capacity is directly proportional to the magnitude of the systemic to pulmonary artery shunt and most limited in patients with the smallest pulmonary blood flow and the largest right-to-left shunt during exercise.[31] Following intracardiac repair, there is

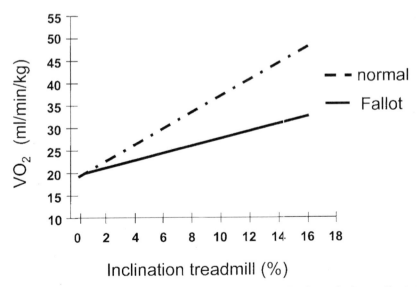

Figure 1. Typical example of the slope of VO_2 versus exercise intensity in a patient after tetralogy repair and a normal control. A steeper curve in normals reflects a higher efficiency of O_2 transport.

marked improvement of work capacity, with an average VO_{2max} reaching 81% of normal,[4] but as pointed out before, reported exercise performance varies considerably between studies. Exercise capacity of postoperative tetralogy patients should probably not be assessed as if they were a single, homogeneous population.[9] The degree of pulmonary artery hypoplasia and RV outflow tract obstruction prior to repair vary widely, and as a result the postoperative residual obstruction and pulmonary regurgitation vary as much. The poorest results of exercise performance after intracardiac repair were found in patients corrected as adults.[32] If patients are corrected in childhood, work capacity appears to be more related to a good surgical outcome than age at intracardiac repair per se.[15]

Heart Rate Response

Heart rate (HR) response during graded exercise and exercise performance tests based on HR response have traditionally been considered to be reliable indicators of the circulatory functional capacity in adults[33] and children[34] with cardiovascular disease. Most exercise studies in patients with corrected tetralogy have shown significantly reduced maximal as well as submaximal exercise HRs, but normal resting HRs.[4,10] Reybrouck et al.[10] performed comparative studies during graded submaximal exercise in two homogenous groups, 11 boys and 8 girls, in the 5- to 8-year age group, operated for tetralogy. Throughout all exercise levels the mean HR values, compared by an analysis of variance (ANOVA), were significantly lower in these patients than in normal children matched for sex, age, body weight, and height. Individual values for HR response during exercise in the 11 boys studied are represented in Figure 2.

Performance indices, which are based on regressing HR on work rate, such as the W170 (power at a HR of 170 beats/min), tend to overestimate work capacity in the presence of a reduced HR response to exercise and should therefore not be used in tetralogy patients.[10,29,35,36] In patients operated for tetralogy, an increased stroke volume does not compensate for the relative bradycardia during exercise, as found in endurance-trained athletes. In these patients stroke volume during exercise has been shown to be considerably lower than in age- and sex-matched healthy subjects,[32,37,38] and consequently cardiac output may be severely reduced[32,37,39,40] and maximal oxygen uptake markedly decreased.[4,32]

The mechanisms underlying the subnormal HR response to exercise have not been clearly defined and appear to be multifactorial.[32,41] Failure to increase HR during exercise has been ascribed to sinus node dysfunction,[10] an impaired function of the autonomic nervous system,[15] a compensatory increase in diastolic filling time, subnormal preload of the right heart during exercise, or the presence of conduction disturbances (e.g., right bundle branch block).[32,42]

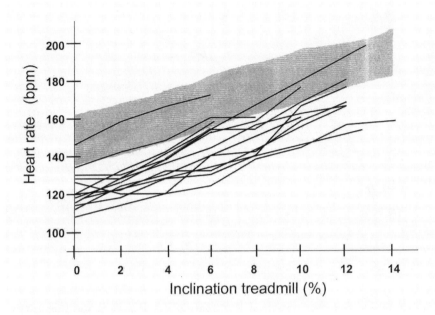

Figure 2. Individual values for heart rate response during graded treadmill exercise in 11 boys (aged 5 to 8 years) operated for tetralogy. The normal range (mean value ± 1 SD) is shown by the *shaded area*.[10]

Most studies have implicated chronotropic impairment as a significant factor in determining aerobic capacity following repair of tetralogy,[10,12,14,43] but this could not be demonstrated by Mulla et al.,[9] who suggested that the main factor limiting aerobic capacity appears to be primarily right-sided cardiac dysfunction rather than chronotropic impairment.

Residual Right Ventricular Outflow Obstruction and Pulmonary Regurgitation

Exercise performance seems to be minimally affected by isolated mild to moderate RV outflow obstruction and similarly, mild pulmonary regurgitation appears to be well tolerated.[4] More severe degrees of pulmonary regurgitation have a deleterious effect though, particularly when associated with RV outflow obstruction or pulmonary branch stenosis.[4] The question of pulmonary regurgitation has been addressed by many studies, due to the controversies surrounding the importance of chronic pulmonary regurgitation in the long term. Most studies (but not all) have demonstrated a significant relationship between the degree of pulmonary regurgitation, abnormal RV function, and decreased exercise capacity.[4]

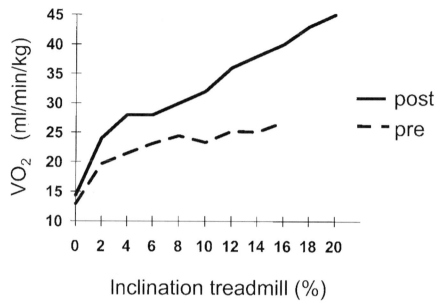

Figure 3. Typical example of the slope of VO$_2$ versus exercise intensity in a patient before and after pulmonary valve replacement for severe pulmonary regurgitation.[17]

Moreover, improved exercise function has well been documented after surgical correction of pulmonary regurgitation with valved conduits.[17,44] A typical example of the slope of VO$_2$ versus exercise intensity in a tetralogy patient before and after pulmonary valve replacement for severe pulmonary regurgitation is shown in Figure 3.

Whereas the indications for intervention are becoming clearer, the optimal time for restoring competence of the RV outflow following previous repair of tetralogy, aiming both for symptomatic improvement and preservation of RV function, should be better defined.[45]

Biventricular Function and Exercise Performance

The introduction of palliation in tetralogy patients by means of construction of a systemic-to-pulmonary shunt in the late 1940s paved the way for the modern management.[46] The operative mortality for surgical correction is currently less than 1% in most centers. Modern techniques for cardiopulmonary bypass and myocardial preservation are important factors facilitating the low perioperative mortality. With improved surgical success, research has become increasingly focused on early and late morbidity, with particular reference to RV function and its relationship to outcome.[46]

Isolated RV restrictive physiology is common after repair of tetralogy.[47,48] The hallmark of isolated RV restriction is laminar antegrade diastolic pulmonary arterial flow coincident with atrial systole, present throughout the respiratory circle.[49] When present in the immediate period after surgical repair, RV restriction is associated with a longer and more troublesome postoperative course.[47] In contrast, the same physiology in the long-term limits pulmonary regurgitation, prevents excessive RV dilatation and, combined with the antegrade pulmonary arterial flow consequent upon atrial contraction, maintains cardiac output, particularly on exercise.[48,50] Multiple factors seem to play a role in the development of restrictive RV physiology, such as cyanosis, obstruction within the RV outflow and pulmonary arterial anatomy, previous palliations, age at repair, and surgical techniques and myocardial protection.[45]

The functional significance of important pulmonary regurgitation after repair of tetralogy and its deleterious effects on RV function and exercise capacity, have been pointed out before. Pulmonary regurgitation seems to affect not only the RV function but also the left ventricular (LV) function under exercise stress.[51] Right ventricular dilatation affects the geometry of the interventricular septum to prevent the LV from appropriately changing shape or accommodating an increased preload during diastolic filling.[52] Moreover, fibrosis or hypertrophy of the septum, induced by chronic overload, could adversely affect systolic function.

Arrhythmias

Impaired exercise capacity and ventricular arrhythmia have been proposed as risk factors for sudden death after repair of tetralogy.[53,54] However, the predisposing factors remain controversial,[55] even though residual hemodynamic abnormalities after surgery,[56,57] age at surgery,[57–59] and duration of follow-up[55,60] are considered crucial. Exercise is superior to routine electrocardiograms (ECGs) in detecting arrhythmias but not as effective as 24-hour ECG monitoring.[4] In exercise studies, arrhythmias are more commonly seen at rest, prior to exercise, and during immediate recovery. The incidence of ventricular arrhythmias with exercise varies greatly between studies, from 0% to as much as 73.3% of patients.[4] During exercise premature ventricular contractions (PVCs) are often reduced in frequency or completely suppressed when the sinus rate approaches or exceeds the PVC rate. Suppression of PVCs during exercise is however of no prognostic significance.[4] Moreover, sustained ventricular tachycardia has been provoked during electrophysiological studies in the absence of any ventricular arrhythmia during exercise.[61,62]

In most previous studies, reports of supraventricular arrhythmias have been less common than that of ventricular arrhythmias.[4] In the most recent study however, 18 of 53 patients (34%), followed on average for 17 years, had SVT, atrial flutter, or atrial fibrillation, suggesting that supraventricular arrhythmias may in the future become more important in adults after repair of tetralogy.[63]

Lung Function and Ventilatory Response to Exercise

The first reports on restrictive lung volume patterns in tetralogy, were in patients who had undergone palliation or repair as adults.[30,64,65] These initial studies showed a reduction of vital capacity (FEV) and total lung capacity of about 25%. FEV and VO_{2max} are linearly related and therefore a significant reduction of FEV should affect maximal work capacity. Several factors may play a role in restrictive lung function, i.e., small lungs due to congenital hypoplasia, altered pulmonary and chest wall mechanics secondary to pulmonary vascular changes, increased pulmonary blood volume, the effects of thoracotomy including scoliosis, and lack of physical activity before and after surgical correction.[4] Patients who underwent intracardiac repair before late adolescence have on average a mild to moderate restrictive ventilatory defect without evidence of airway obstruction.[4] In patients with an excellent surgical outcome and especially without pulmonary regurgitation, lung volumes and capacities may be entirely normal after repair, with or without prior palliation.[16] In studies reporting lung function data as part of exercise evaluation, the lowest FEV% and work performance was found in patients with significant cardiomegaly or pulmonary regurgitation and in patients with significant scoliosis.[4]

Tetralogy patients without any surgical correction or with only shunt palliation hyperventilate at rest and have an increased ventilatory response to exercise.[29,31,65,66] Progressive hypoxemia[66] and an increased ventilation perfusion (VA/Q) mismatch have been suggested as possible explanations for the hyperventilation in these patients. Although patients may have a normal ventilatory response to exercise after repair, a persistent increased ventilatory response to exercise after tetralogy repair has been well documented,[36,50,67] even though these patients are no longer hypoxemic at rest or with exercise. This could be explained by a persistent VA/Q mismatch[68] and/or the inability to increase pulmonary blood flow appropriately with exercise.[50]

Physical Training and Improved Exercise Performance

Because of chronic physical inactivity before and also after surgical correction of tetralogy, physical training may be beneficial to patients after intracardiac repair.[4] The importance of physical activity has been supported by subsequent training studies after repair, which all showed improved physical performance after training,[69-72] and by observations that patients who participate in varsity sports after repair perform better than patient with a sedentary life style.[15,41]

Conclusions

Over the previous four decades, the management of patients with tetralogy has evolved considerably, with numerous advances in the technique and timing of repair. Throughout this evolution age at repair and surgical technique have been intimately related.[73] Most patients have an excellent functional result after intracardiac repair and lead a normal active and social life.[1-3] With improved surgical success, research has become increasingly focused on early and late morbidity, with particular reference to RV function and its relationship to outcome.[46]

Exercise testing should be an integral part of the long-term evaluation of tetralogy after surgical correction, as subjective (self-reporting) estimates of activity level are poorly associated with objective measurements of exercise capacity.[7] Attempts should be made to standardize exercise testing in patients with congenital heart disease, so that a greater uniformity can be developed with regard to methodology, as well as data presentation.[4]

There has been uniform agreement that, as a group, patients with repaired tetralogy have mild to moderate reduction in aerobic capacity, although individual variations are large. Long-standing significant pulmonary regurgitation has been shown to be associated with RV dysfunction, ventricular arrhythmias and impaired exercise tolerance. Improvement of aerobic capacity after surgical correction of pulmonary regurgitation with implantation of valved conduits has been well documented.[17,44]

Restrictive RV diastolic physiology seems to prevent excessive RV dilatation, preserving exercise capacity and decreasing the risk of malignant ventricular arrhythmias.[48,50]

Appropriate physical training after surgical repair of tetralogy may be beneficial to patients and has shown to improve exercise tolerance.[4]

References

1. Katz NM, Blackstone EH, Kirklin JW, et al. Late survival and symptoms after repair of tetralogy of Fallot. *Circulation* 1982;65:405–410.
2. Murphy JG, Gersch BJ, Phil D, et al. Long-term outcome in patients undergoing surgical repair of tetralogy of Fallot. *N Engl J Med* 1993;329:593–599.
3. Nollert G, Fischlein T, Bouterwek S, et al. Long-term survival in patients with repair of tetralogy of Fallot: 36-year follow-up of 490 survivors of the first year after surgical repair. *J Am Coll Cardiol* 1997;5:1374–1383.
4. Wessel HU, Paul MH. Exercise studies in tetralogy of Fallot: A review. *Pediatr Cardiol* 1999;20:39–47.

5. Klesges RC, Eck LH, Mellon MW, et al. The accuracy of self-reports of physical activity. *Med Sci Sports Exerc* 1990;22:690–697.
6. Jones NL. Clinical Exercise Testing. Philidelphia: WB Saunders, 1988:9–12.
7. Rogers R, Reybrouck T, Weymans M, et al. Reliability of subjective estimates of exercise capacity after total repair of tetralogy of Fallot. *Acta Paediatr* 1994;83:866–869.
8. LaPorte RE, Montoye HS, Caspersen CJ. Assessment of physical activity in epidemiological research; problems and prospects. *Public Health Rep* 1985; 100:131–146.
9. Mulla N, Simpson P, Sullivan NM, et al. Determinants of aerobic capacity during exercise following complete repair of tetralogy of Fallot with a transannular patch. *Pediatr Cardiol* 1997;18:350–356.
10. Reybrouck T, Weymans M, Stijns H, et al. Exercise testing after correction of tetralogy of fallot: the fallacy of a reduced heart rate response. *Am Heart J* 1986;112:958–1003.
11. Horneffer PJ, Zahka KG, Rowe SA, et al. Long-term results of total repair of tetralogy of Fallot in childhood. *Am Thorac Surg* 1990;50:179–185.
12. Lambert J, Ferguson RJ, Gervais A, et al. Exercise capacity, residual abnormalities and activity habits following total correction for tetralogy of Fallot. *Cardiology* 1980;66:120–131.
13. Rowe SA, Zahka KG, Manolio TA, et al. Lung function and pulmonary regurgitation limit exercise capacity in postoperative tetralogy of Fallot. *J Am Coll Cardiol* 1991;17:461–466.
14. Takkunen O, Mattila S, Nieminen MS, et al. Cardiorespiratory function after correction of tetralogy of Fallot. *Scan J Thorac Cardiovasc Surg* 1987;21:21–26.
15. Wessel HU, Cunningham WJ, Paul MH, et al. Lung function in tetralogy of Fallot after intracardiac repair. *J Thorac Cardiovasc Surg* 1980;80:582–593.
16. Wessel HU, Weiner MD, Paul MH, et al. Lung function in tetralogy of Fallot after intracardiac repair. *J Thorac Cardiovasc Surg* 1981;82:416–428.
17. Eyskens B, Reybrouck T, Bogaert J, et al. Homograft insertion for pulmonary regurgitation after repair of tetralogy of Fallot improves cardiorespiratory exercise performance. *Am J Cardiol* 2000;85:221–225.
18. Sarubbi B, Pacileo G, Pisacane C, et al. Exercise capacity in young patients after total repair of tetralogy of Fallot. *Pediatr Cardiol* 2000;21:211–215.
19. Beaver WL, Wasserman K, Whipp BJ. A new method for detecting anaerobic threshold by gas exchange. *J Appl Physiol* 1986;60:2020–2027.
20. Reybrouck T, Deroost F, Van Der Hauwaert LG. Evaluation of breath-by-breath measurement of respiratory gas exchange in pediatric exercise testing. *Chest* 1992;102:147–152.
21. Reybrouck T, Mertens L, Kalis N, et al. Dynamics of respiratory gas exchange during exercise after correction of congenital heart disease. *J Appl Physiol* 1996;80:458–463.
22. Wasserman K, Beaver WL, Whipp BJ. Gas exchange theory and the lactic acidosis (anaerobic) threshold. *Circulation* 1990;81(suppl II):II-14–30.
23. Reybrouck T, Weymans M, Stijns H, et al. Ventilatory anaerobic threshold in healthy children: Age and sex differences. *Eur J Appl Physiol* 1985;54:278–284.
24. Cabrera ME, Chizeck HJ. On the existence of a lactate threshold during incremental exercise: A systems analysis. *J Appl Physiol* 1996;80:1819–1828.
25. Shimizu M, Myers J, Buchanan N, et al. The ventilatory threshold: Method protocol and evaluator agreement. *Am Heart J* 1991;122:509–516.
26. Meyer K, Hajric R, Westbrook S, et al. Ventilatory and lactate threshold determinations in healthy normals and cardiac patients: Methodological problems. *Eur J Appl Physiol* 1996;72:387–393.

27. Cohen-Solal A, Chabernaud JM, Gourgon R. Comparison of oxygen uptake during bicycle exercise in patients with chronic heart failure and normal subjects. *J Am Coll Cardiol* 1990;16:80–85.

28. Hansen JE, DY S, Oren A, et al. Relation of oxygen uptake to work rate in normal men and men with circulatory disorders. *Am J Cardiol* 1987;59:669–674.

29. Crawford DW, Simpson E, McIlroy MB. Cardiopulmonary function in Fallot's tetralogy after palliative shunting operations. *Am Heart J* 1967;74:463–472.

30. Bjarke B. Spirometric data, pulmonary ventilation and gas exchange at rest and during exercise in adult patients with tetralogy of Fallot. *Scand J Resp Dis* 1974;55:47–61.

31. Gold WM, Mattioli LF, Price AC. Response to exercise in patients with tetralogy of Fallot with systemic-pulmonary anastomoses. *Pediatrics* 1969;43:781–793.

32. Bjarke B. Oxygen uptake and cardiac output during maximal and submaximal exercise in adult subjects with totally corrected tetralogy of Fallot. *Scand J Thorac Cardiovasc Surg* 1974;16(Suppl):1–29.

33. Mitchell JH, Blomqvist CG. Response of patients with heart disease to dynamic and static exercise. In: Pollock ML, Schmidt DH, (eds). *Heart disease and rehabilitation*. Boston: Houghton Mifflin Professional Publishers, 1979, pp. 86.

34. Duffie ER, Adams FH. The use of the working capacity test in the evaluation of children with congenital heart disease. *Pediatrics* 1963;32(suppl):757–768.

35. Mocellin R, Bastanier CK. Frage der Zuverlassigkeit der W170 als Mass der korperlichen Leistungsfahigkeit bei Beurteilung von Kindern mit Herzkrankheiten. *Eur J Pediatr* 1976;122:223–239.

36. Wessel HU. Integrated cardiopulmonary approach to exercise testing. *Pediatrician* 1986;13:26–33.

37. Epstein SE, Beiser DG, Goldstein RE, et al. Hemodynamic abnormalities in response to mild and intense upright exercise following operative correction of an atrial septal defect or tetralogy of Fallot. *Circulation* 1973;47:1065–1075.

38. Hirschfeld S, Tubolen-metzger AJ, Borkat G, et al. Comparison of exercise and catheterisation results following total surgical correction of tetralogy of Fallot. *J Thorac Cardiovasc Surg* 1978;75:446–451.

39. Cumming GR. Maximal supine exercise hemodynamics after open heart surgery for Fallot's tetralogy. *Br Heart J* 1979;41:683–691.

40. Rocchini AP. Hemodynamic abnormalities in response to supine exercise in patients after operative correction of tetralogy of Fallot after early childhood. *Am J Cardiol* 1981;48:325–330.

41. James FW, Kaplan S, Schwartz DC, et al. Response to exercise in patients after total correction of tetralogy of Fallot. *Circulation* 1976;54:671–679.

42. Rigolin VH, Li JS, Hanson MW, et al. The role of right ventricular and pulmonary functional abnormalities in limiting exercise capacity in adults with congenital heart disease. *Am J Cardiol* 1997;80:315–322.

43. Paridon SM. Exercise response in tetralogy of Fallot and pulmonary atresia with ventricular septal defect. *Prog Pediatr Cardiol* 1993;2:35–43.

44. Warner KG, Anderson JE, Fulton DR, et al. Restoration of the pulmonary valve reduces right ventricular volume overload after previous repair of tetralogy of Fallot. *Circulation* 1993;88:II 189–197.

45. Gatzoulis MA. Is the pulmonary valve important in repaired tetralogy of Fallot? In: Redington AN, Brawn WJ, Deanfield JE, Anderson RH, (eds). *The Right Heart in Congenital Heart Disease*. London: Greenwich Medical Media Ltd, 199, pp. 85–89.

46. Cullen S. The right ventricle in tetralogy of Fallot: The early postoperative period. In: Redington AN, Brawn WJ, Deanfield JE, Anderson RH, (eds). *The Right*

Heart in Congenital Heart Disease. London: Greenwich Medical Media Ltd, 1998, pp. 81–84.

47. Cullen S, Shore DF, Redington AN. Characterisation of right ventricular diastolic performance after complete repair of tetralogy of Fallot: Restrictive physiology predicts slow postoperative recovery. *Circulation* 1995;91:1782–1789.

48. Gatzoulis MA, Clark AL, Cullen S, et al. Right ventricular diastolic function 15 to 35 years after repair of tetralogy of Fallot: Restrictive physiology predicts superior exercise performance. *Circulation* 1995;91:1775–1781.

49. Gatzoulis MA, Norgard G, Redington AN. Biventricular long axis function after repair of tetralogy of Fallot. *Pediatr Cardiol* 1998;19:128–132.

50. Clark AL, Gatzoulis MA, Redington AN. Ventilatory responses to exercise in adults after repair of tetralogy of Fallot. *Br Heart J* 1995;73:445–449.

51. Kondo C, Nakazawa M, Kusakabe K, et al. Left ventricular dysfunction on exercise long term after total repair of tetralogy of Fallot. *Circulation* 1995;92(suppl II):II-250–5.

52. Pearlman AS, Clark CE, Henry WL, et al. Determinants of ventricular septal motion: Influence of relative right and left ventricular size. *Circulation* 1976;54:83–91.

53. Garson A, Nihil MR, McNamara DG, et al. Status of the adult and adolescent after repair of tetralogy of Fallot. *Circulation* 1979;59:1232–1240.

54. Quattlebaum TG, Varghese PJ, Neill CA, et al. Sudden death among postoperative patients with tetralogy of Fallot: A follow-up study of 243 patients for an average of twelve years. *Circulation* 1976;54:289–293.

55. Deanfield JE. Late ventricular arrhythmia occurring after repair of tetralogy of Fallot. Do they matter? *Int J Cardiol* 1991;30:143–150.

56. Kavey RW, Thomas FD, Byrum CJ, et al. Ventricular arrhythmia and biventricular dysfunction after repair of tetralogy of Fallot. *J Am Coll Cardiol* 1984;4:126–131.

57. Kobayashi J, Hirose H, Nakano S, et al. Ambulatory electrocardiographic study of the frequency and cause of ventricular arrhythmia after correction of tetralogy of Fallot. *Am J Cardiol* 1984;54:1310–1313.

58. Deanfield JE, McKenna WJ, Presbitero P, et al. Ventricular arrhythmia in unrepaired and repaired tetralogy of Fallot: Relation to age, timing of repair, and haemodynamic status. *Br Heart J* 1984;52:77–81.

59. Garson A, Randall DC, Gilette PC, et al. Prevention of sudden death after repair of tetralogy of Fallot. *J Am Coll Cardiol* 1985;6:221–227.

60. Vaksmann G, Rounier A, Davignon A, et al. Frequency and prognosis of arrhythmia after operative 'correction' of tetralogy of Fallot. *Am J Cardiol* 1990;66:346–349.

61. Dunningan A, Pritzger MR, Benditt DG, et al. Life threatening ventricular tachycardia in late survivors of surgically corrected tetralogy of Fallot. *Br Heart J* 1984;52:198–206.

62. Kugler JD, Pinsky WW, Cheatham JP, et al. Sustained ventricular tachycardia after repair of tetralogy of Fallot: New electrophysiologic findings. *Am J Cardiol* 1983;51:1137–1143.

63. Roos-Hesselink J, Perlroth MG, McGhie J, et al. Atrial arrhythmias in adults after repair of tetralogy of Fallot. Correlations with clinical, exercise and echocardiographic findings. *Circulation* 1995;91:2214–2219.

64. Strieder DJ, Aziz KU, Zaver AG, et al. Exercise tolerance after repair of tetralogy of Fallot. *Ann Thorac Surg* 1975;19:397–405.

65. Strieder DJ, Mesko ZG, Aziz K. Respiratory control and exercise ventilation in tetralogy of Fallot. *Acta Pediatr Belgium* 1974;28(Suppl):162–168.

66. Taylor MR. The ventilatory response to hypoxia during exercise in cyanotic congenital heart disease. *Clin Sci* 1973;45:99–105.
67. Grant GP, Garofano RP, Mansell AL, et al. Ventilatory response to exercise after intracardiac repair of tetralogy of Fallot. *Am Rev Respir Dis* 1992;144:833–836.
68. Goldberg SJ. Functional evaluation of children with congenital heart disease by response to maximal exercise. *UCLA Forum Med Sci* 1970;10:295–304.
69. Bradley LM, Galioto FM Jr, Vaccaro P, et al. Effect of intense aerobic training on exercise performance in children after surgical repair of tetralogy of Fallot or complete transposition of the great arteries. *Am J Cardiol* 1985;56:816–818.
70. Calzolari A, Turchetta A, Biondi G, et al. Rehabilitation of children after total correction of tetralogy of Fallot. *Int J Cardiol* 1990;28:151–158.
71. Goldberg B, Fripp RR, Lister G, et al. Effect of physical training on exercise performance of children following surgical repair of congenital heart disease. *Pediatrics* 1981;68:691–699.
72. Ruttenberg HD, Adams TD, Orsmond GS, et al. Defects of exercise training on aerobic fitness in children after open heart surgery. *Pediatr Cardiol* 1983;4:19–24.
73. McElhinney DB, Parry AJ, Reddy VM, et al. Tetralogy of Fallot: When is the optimal time for repair? In: Redington AN, Brawn WJ, Deanfield JE, Anderson RH, (eds). *The Right Heart in Congenital Heart Disease*. London: Greenwich Medical Media Ltd, 1998, pp. 75–80.

Chapter IV

Right Ventricular Function and Pulmonary Regurgitation in Postoperative Tetralogy of Fallot

Thomas P. Graham, Jr.

Introduction

The assessment of right ventricular (RV) function in patients with congenital heart disease is an important aspect of optimal long-term follow-up of many postoperative patients, including those with transposition of the great arteries, tetralogy of Fallot and single right ventricle following Fontan repair. The postoperative tetralogy patient is a major case in point where the repetitive assessment of RV function is essential for effective clinical management.

Despite the excellent clinical outcome of most adults with repaired tetralogy of Fallot,[1] many patients have varying degrees of moderate pulmonary regurgitation that can be difficult to quantify. In addition, pulmonary artery stenosis, tricuspid regurgitation, left ventricular (LV) dysfunction, and even mild increases in pulmonary vascular resistance can complicate evaluation of the effects of pulmonary regurgitation per se on RV function.

One of the most perplexing and unresolved questions in adult congenital heart disease is when to intervene in terms of replacement of the pulmonary valve in postoperative tetralogy patients with significant volume overload secondary to pulmonary regurgitation. Although the operative mortality is extremely low,[2] the long-term durability of the pulmonary valve and the questions as to whether or not valve replacement will enhance longevity, improve ventricular function, and improve quality of life are unanswered and complicate this decision making process.

The purpose of this monograph is to define an approach for the clini-

From Gatzoulis MA, Murphy DJ (eds): *The Adult with Tetralogy of Fallot: The ISACCD Monograph Series* ©Futura Publishing Co., Inc, Armonk, NY, 2001.

cal and laboratory assessment of RV function and pulmonary regurgitation in tetralogy patients and to put this in the context of management decisions regarding pulmonary valve replacement.

Variables Associated with Right Ventricular Dysfunction Post Tetralogy Repair

The important variables associated with RV dysfunction post tetralogy repair are listed in Table 1. Of particular importance is RV hypertension, which can be caused by anatomical obstruction at the valve annulus, above the valve, or at the infundibular level. In addition, those patients who have had a prior conduit or homograft used for repair can have anatomical obstruction at the site of insertion into the ventricle or pulmonary artery or can develop an obstructive intimal peel.

Another potential cause of RV hypertension is pulmonary artery stenosis, usually left pulmonary artery obstruction at the site of the former ductus insertion or sometimes at the site of a previous shunt. Finally, pulmonary hypertension can be present in some older patients who had a large aorto-pulmonary shunt that was present for a considerable period of time before repair. In addition, there could be pulmonary hypertension secondary to pulmonary venous or mitral level obstruction, LV diastolic pressure elevation, or intrinsic pulmonary disease such as severe kyphoscoliosis.

Chronic valvular regurgitation per se will affect ventricular function; the deleterious effects of chronic left sided regurgitation on LV function are

---

Table 1.
Variables Associated with Right Ventricular Dysfunction Post Tetralogy Repair.

Right Ventricular Hypertension:
   Right ventricular outflow obstruction: annular, supravalvular, infundibular
   Conduit/Homograft obstruction
   Pulmonary artery obstruction left > right
   Pulmonary Hypertension: arterial, pulmonary venous or left heart obstruction, pulmonary disease
Valvular Regurgitation:
   Pulmonary regurgitation: markedly increased by pulmonary artery hypertension
   Tricuspid regurgitation
Other Right Ventricular Hemodynamic/Anatomical Abnormalities:
   Right ventricular outflow incision/scar—akinesia
   Right ventricular outflow patch: akinesia
   Right ventricular outflow aneurysmal dilatation: dyskinesia
Right and Left Ventricular Myocardial Abnormalities:
   Secondary to inadequate intraoperative myocardial protection and/or reperfusion injury
   Secondary to preoperative pressure overload
   Secondary to preoperative cyanosis

well documented.[3] One of the most striking examples of the effects of volume overload on the right ventricle is a report of the natural history of isolated pulmonary valve incompetence.[4] In this review of reported cases,[4] almost half of the patients with this condition had become symptomatic by age 40 (Figure 1).

The effect of pure pulmonary regurgitation in an individual patient is shown in Figure 2. These films were taken at 2 years and 14 years in a boy who had pulmonary valvectomy at age 3 months. There is massive cardiomegaly which developed in the intervening 12 years between films, which was associated with symptoms of easy fatiguability. At age 14, he had severe pulmonary regurgitation, massive RV enlargement, and an RV pressure of 30/6. Successful pulmonary valve replacement resulted in an improvement in symptoms and a decrease in heart size to the same cardiothoracic ratio that was present at age 2 years.

In addition to pulmonary regurgitation, tricuspid regurgitation can also be a cause of (or an effect of) RV enlargement and dysfunction. With pulmonary valve replacement and a decrease in RV volume, tricuspid regurgitation usually will decrease significantly. The decision as to whether or not to perform a tricuspid valvuloplasty or replacement at the time of pulmonary valve replacement when both valves are incompetent is a difficult one, and usually made in the operating room with the aid of transesophageal echocardiography.

In addition to these valvular abnormalities there are abnormalities related to the surgery itself including the RV outflow incision and scar, which results in a sizeable akinetic area of the RV chamber. The scar will

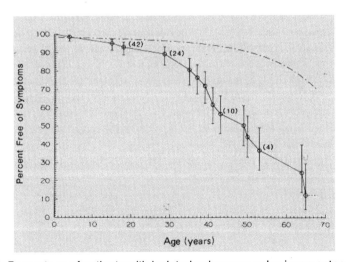

Figure 1. Percentage of patients with isolated pulmonary valve incompetence free of symptoms as a function of age (by permission).[4]

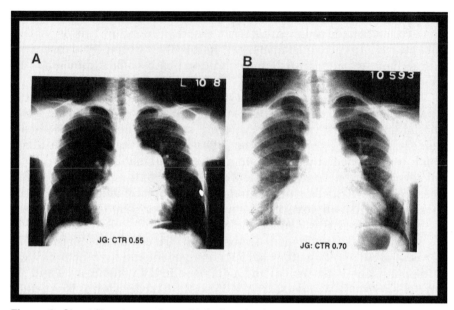

Figure 2. Chest films in a patient with isolated pulmonary valve incompetence at age 2 years (left panel) and 14 years (right panel) demonstrated a marked increase in heart size between films.

grow with growth of the heart and can be quite sizable even in a patient who had surgery early in life. In addition, the RV outflow patch will be akinetic and may be oversized leading to significant "dead space" in this area. Further, there can be aneurysmal dilation of the outflow tract and main pulmonary artery leading to dyskinesia affecting RV function.

Finally, there can be RV and/or LV myocardial abnormalities secondary to inadequate intraoperative myocardial protection and/or reperfusion injury. This is particularly important in older patients since they will not have had the advantage of current methods of attempting to optimize myocardial protection and reperfusion injury. In addition, there can be myocardial abnormalities secondary to preoperative pressure overload and cyanosis which are known to be more significant in patients who have had repair at an older age.

Clinical Assessment (Table 2)

History

The patient's history may frequently underestimate the severity of RV dysfunction or pulmonary regurgitation. Many patients will indicate that they have no symptoms, but will be unable to perform in a satisfactory

Table 2.
**Clinical Assessment of Right Ventricular Function and
Pulmonary Regurgitation.**

History:
  Frequently underestimates the severity
  Fatiguability—assess for depression, sedentary lifestyle
  Exercise intolerance
  Arrhythmia
  Lung-disease, chest deformity, asthma
  Smoking, substance abuse
Physical Exam:
  Right ventricular parasternal lift—can be misleadingly normal in adults with thick
    chest
  Pulmonary Regurgitation murmur:
    Intensity and duration correlate fairly well with severity.
    Differentiate from aortic regurgitation: pulmonary regurgitation lower frequency
      and heard better with bell of the stethoscope unless pulmonary hypertension
      present
  Evaluate jugular venous pulsation
  Evaluate for hepatomegaly, edema, ascites

manner with formal exercise testing. Easy fatiguability, an important sign of RV dysfunction and/or pulmonary regurgitation, must be considered in the light of other potential causes of this common complaint, such as depression or sedentary life style. Exercise intolerance needs to be quantified with exercise testing as discussed below and in Chapter III. Arrhythmia can be a marker for serious ventricular dysfunction and/or severe volume overload. Patients with symptomatic arrhythmia should be evaluated without delay.

Lung disease, chest deformity such as kyphoscoliosis, or asthma all can enhance pulmonary regurgitation and RV dysfunction and should be considered in the history. Finally, smoking and substance abuse should be evaluated as these can both affect ventricular function.

Physical Examination

Patients with significant pulmonary regurgitation usually will have a significant RV parasternal lift. Palpation, however, can be misleadingly normal in adults with a thick chest wall and/or an increased anterior-posterior diameter. The pulmonary regurgitant murmur, in general, will reflect severity reasonably well. Increased intensity and duration generally correlate with more severe regurgitation. Pulmonary regurgitation must be differentiated from aortic regurgitation, since this condition also can occur in adults post tetralogy repair. Most pulmonary regurgitant murmurs are heard best with the bell of the stethoscope, unless significant pulmonary hypertension is present. Aortic regurgitation and pulmonary regurgitation in the presence of severe pulmonary hypertension will be heard best with the diaphragm. The jugular venous pulsation usually will be a reliable indicator of any increase in filling pressure of the right side and should always be evaluated carefully. Liver enlargement and peripheral edema will be present when RV failure has ensued.

Laboratory Assessment: ECG (Table 3)

Most patients will have sinus rhythm and right bundle branch block. If tachycardia is present, one should carefully evaluate the ECG for an atrial arrhythmia with or without variable AV block, since this rhythm could precipitate cardiac decompensation.

In the presence of right bundle branch block, the characterization of RV hypertrophy is not possible. Right atrial enlargement gives an indication of elevated RV filling pressure and/or tricuspid regurgitation. An increased QRS duration has been reported as indicative of the severity of RV enlargement.[5,6] This finding appears to be more useful in patients with a marked interval increase in QRS duration. Many patients, however, have only modest increases in QRS duration even in the presence of severe pulmonary regurgitation.

Ambulatory ECG recordings and exercise testing are useful in patients investigated for possible arrhythmia.

Laboratory Assessment: Basic Radiology Studies (Table 4)

The chest film can be quite useful to separate those patients who are very unlikely to have significant pulmonary regurgitation or RV dysfunction from patients who are very likely to have significant RV dysfunction and/or pulmonary regurgitation. If one has excluded significant LV enlargement, a patient with a cardiothoracic-ratio of < 0.50 is unlikely to have significant pulmonary regurgitation, whereas a ratio of > 0.55 is frequently associated with moderate to severe pulmonary regurgitation.

The chest film is also useful to assess for pulmonary disease such as kyphoscoliosis, emphysema, or pulmonary fibrosis. There is also the ability to assess pulmonary artery size with the right frequently larger than the left; a small left pulmonary artery frequently is an indication of left pulmonary

---

Table 3.
Laboratory Assessment: ECG.

RBBB in most—usually not helpful in assessment of right ventricular hypertrophy
QRS duration—? indicative of severity of right ventricular enlargement
Ambulatory ECG/exercise testing useful if symptoms of ? arrhythmia

Table 4.
Laboratory Assessment: Basic Radiology Studies.

Chest x-ray:
    CTR useful to estimate the degree of pulmonary regurgitation (if left ventricular enlargement excluded):
    CTR < 0.50—very unlikely to have significant pulmonary regurgitation
    CTR > 0.55—very likely to have significant pulmonary regurgitation
    Assess for pulmonary disease, Kyphoscoliosis
    Assess for discrepancy in pulmonary artery size: right > left—? left pulmonary artery stenosis
    Assess for main pulmonary artery/right ventricular outflow enlargement
Flow studies:
    Quantify right vs left lung flow
    If discrepant, catheterize to try to dilate/stent left/right pulmonary artery and normalize flow, ? partially unload the right ventricle

artery stenosis. In addition, the x-ray can be used for assessment of significant enlargement of the main pulmonary artery and RV outflow tract area. If there is any question of disparity of flow or pulmonary artery size, it is useful to quantify right versus left lung flow. In the presence of pulmonary artery stenosis, there is frequently a marked increase in percentage of flow to the contralateral lung. These data can indicate a need for cardiac catheterization to try to dilate and stent the stenotic pulmonary artery to normalize flow and decrease the pressure and secondary volume load on the right ventricle.

Laboratory Assessment: Echocardiography - Doppler Studies (Table 5)

Echocardiography, as in all congenital cardiac abnormalities is quite useful. Qualitative assessment of right and LV size and function is usually possible; LV ejection fraction can be determined in most patients, and RV ejection fraction (RVEF) can be measured in some. Right ventricular area change with systole may be useful as a semi-quantitative measure of function in patients in whom good biplane views of the ventricle are not possible. In those patients who have excellent images with transthoracic echo and in whom 3-Dimensional echo is available, RVEF can be quantified.[6,7] Unfortunately, this modality is useful in a small minority of adult patients since it is not available in most centers at the present time and adequate images for its use are rarely found in adults after tetralogy repair. An assessment of the main pulmonary artery, right pulmonary artery, and left pulmonary size is useful as is the evaluation of the tricuspid valve annulus and aortic root size.

Doppler evaluation of pulmonary regurgitation[8] is an important part of the assessment. These studies, however, frequently overestimate the clinical severity of pulmonary regurgitation. If there is reflux from distal

Table 5.
Echocardiographic—Doppler Studies.

Anatomical details:
  Right and left ventricular size
  Qualitative functional assessment
  Left ventricular ejection fraction (LVEF)
  RVEF or area % change
  Main and right/left pulmonary artery size
  Tricuspid valve annulus
  Aortic Root size
Doppler:
  Pulmonary regurgitation:
    Frequently overestimates clinical severity
    Scales of reflux from main and right/left pulmonary artery into right ventricle
  Right ventricular obstruction: annular, infundibular, valvular, conduit
  Pulmonary artery stenosis
  Tricuspid regurgitation
  Aortic regurgitation
  Myocardial Performance Index
  Diastolic function

main pulmonary artery or from right or left pulmonary artery back into the RV outflow tract or body of the right ventricle, this generally indicates severe pulmonary regurgitation.

Pulmonary artery stenosis can generally be quantified with Doppler estimations if adequate views are available. In addition, tricuspid and aortic regurgitation should be assessed and the tricuspid regurgitation jet should be used to estimate RV pressure. The myocardial performance index,[9] seen in Figure 3, is a simple calculation which can be useful to follow patients. Its utility in predicting outcome is not known at present.

Right ventricular diastolic dysfunction has been reported in postoperative tetralogy patients who demonstrated forward diastolic flow in the pulmonary artery coincident with atrial systole[10] (see Figure 4). These patients have also shown superior vena caval reversal with atrial systole and short transtricuspid E-wave deceleration time; such findings are consistent with a stiff right ventricle acting as a conduit between right atrium and pulmonary artery.[10] Interestingly, these patients usually have smaller right ventricles, less pulmonary regurgitation, and better exercise performance than their counterparts without restrictive physiology.[10]

Laboratory Assessment: Exercise Studies (Table 6)

Exercise studies are helpful in patients in whom severity of RV dysfunction and pulmonary regurgitation are not clearly evident from other studies. Treadmill studies are more commonly used than bicycle studies and normal parameters for age and sex are available. Exercise testing is most use-

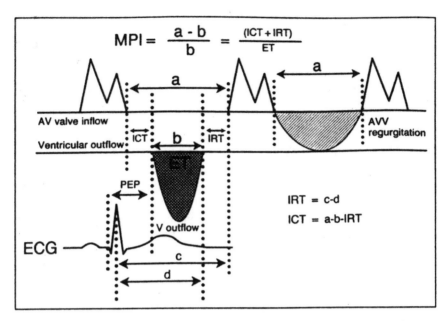

Figure 3. Myocardial performance index calculation (by permission).[9]

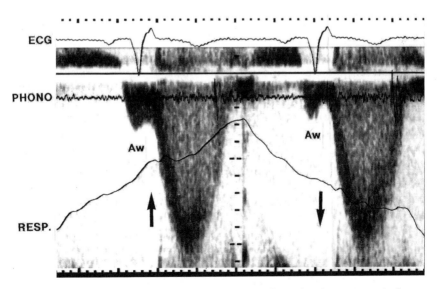

Figure 4. Doppler examination of pulmonary arterial flow showing antegrade flow co-incident with atrial systole (by permission).[10]

Table 6.
Exercise Studies.

Treadmill more commonly used than bicycle: normal parameters for age and sex
Measure VO_2
Measure anaerobic threshold
? Repeat after exercise rehab program if exercise data do not correlate with history,
  clinical assessment

---

ful when VO_2 is measured, anaerobic threshold is determined, and the tests are performed in a facility where these measurements are made on a regular basis with standardized protocols. If there are questions regarding the degree of fitness, these studies should be repeated after an exercise rehabilitation program to enhance exercise ability. The degree of pulmonary regurgitation correlates reasonably well with exercise ability;[11,13] pulmonary valve replacement generally results in improved exercise performance.[12,13]

Laboratory Assessment: Nuclear Cardiology (Table 7)

Nuclear cardiology studies can be performed in centers where there is experience and expertise in these procedures (Table 7). Both first pass and equilibrium studies have been used. Equilibrium studies are more commonly used now. The large right atrium present in many of these patients can result in underestimation of RVEF by the equilibrium technique. One of the important characteristics of the nuclear cardiology studies is that the rest and exercise studies can be performed with RVEF measured at both states.[14] The patient with a normal RV response should increase by 5% or more in ejection fraction units with adequate exercise. It is important to have local expertise and normal data for one's own lab to use these studies effectively. Many nuclear laboratories do not routinely measure RVEF.

Laboratory Assessment: Magnetic Resonance Imaging Studies (Tables 8&9)

Magnetic resonance imaging (MRI) studies are excellent for assessing the size and the anatomical details of the pulmonary arteries, the aorta, RV and LV relative size, and for qualitative assessment of function. It is also

---

Table 7.
Nuclear Cardiology Studies.

Can measure RVEF, LVEF: 1st pass, equilibrium studies
With large right atrium, equilibrium studies frequently underestimate RVEF
Can determine RVEF with exercise
Must have local expertise and normal data to be useful

Table 8.
MRI Studies.

Excellent for size of main and right/left pulmonary arteries, Aorta, right and left ventricular relative size
Good for pulmonary artery stenoses
Excellent for qualitative assessment of function
Excellent for RVEF/LVEF if local expertise/experience available
Normal values available for ejection fraction and volumes [15,16]

excellent for RV and LV volume, mass and ejection fraction quantitation if local expertise and experience is available, which is not the case in many centers (Figure 5).[15,16] The best normal values for ventricular size and ejection fraction are provided by MRI as indicated in Table 9. When MRI is not

Table 9.
Normal MRI Valves for Adult Volumes and Ejection Fractions.[16]

	Right Ventricle	Left Ventricle
End-diastolic volume (ml/m^2)	75 ± 13	$66 + 12$
(95% Con Lim)	(49–101)	(44–89)
Ejection Fraction (%)	61 ± 7	67 ± 5
	(47–76)	(57–78)

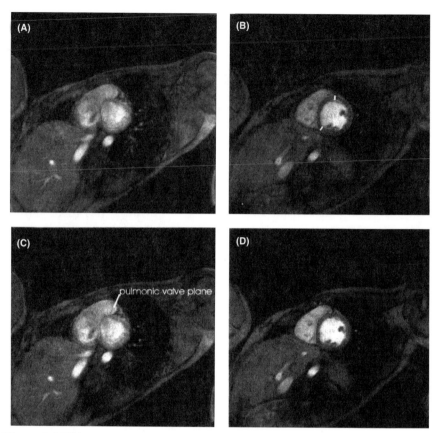

Figure 5. MRI images used to determine right and left ventricular borders and calculate areas for volume determinations (by permission).[16]

feasible because of a pacemaker or other considerations, ultrafast CT can be used to provide similar images.

Laboratory Assessment: Cardiac Catheterization/Angiography (Table 10)

Despite all of these studies, the current gold standard in most centers for measurement of pressures, evaluation of stenoses, and RV function is catheterization. This is particularly important if one has found discrepancy in flow between right and left lung and pulmonary artery stenosis that can be dilated and stented to improve the patient's anatomical condition prior to consideration for pulmonary valve replacement. If an effective dilatation is performed and flow is normalized in terms of distribution to

Table 10.
Cardiac Catheterization/Angiography.

Still "Gold Standard" for pressures, stenoses, Right ventricular function, pulmonary artery anatomy, but echo/MRI combination can yield most of the important data for management

Frequently necessary to diagnose and dilate/stent pulmonary artery stenoses

Table 11.
Indicators for Pulmonary Valve Replacement.

Fatigue, exercise intolerance unexplained by factors other than right ventricular abnormalities

Greater than mild right ventricular enlargement: physical exam, chest x-ray, echo, MRI

Abnormal exercise test: $\downarrow$ VO$_2$ unexplained by other factors

Mild or borderline decreased right ventricular systolic function

Arrhythmia unexplained by factors other than right ventricular enlargement

right and left lungs, it can be useful to reevaluate RV size function as well as exercise ability to determine if the improvement is enough to warrant delaying surgery.

Indicators for Pulmonary Valve Replacement (Table 11)

The final determination, in terms of when to intervene for pulmonary valve replacement despite all of the available studies, can be difficult. Those patients with moderate to severe RV enlargement and moderate to severe pulmonary regurgitation with symptoms, clearly need to have their valve replaced; if they have reached this stage, one has probably waited a bit too long. Because there is a good operation with low morbidity and mortality and the longevity for current bioprosthetic valves is reasonably good, earlier intervention is probably the proper choice. In most patients with border-line decreases in ejection fraction, moderate or greater degrees of pulmonary regurgitation, and modest or greater degrees of exercise intolerance, replacement of the pulmonary valve is indicated.

References

1. Murphy JG, Gersh BJ, Phil D, et al. Long-term outcome in patients undergoing surgical repair of tetralogy of Fallot. *N Engl J Med* 1993;329:593–599.
2. Yemets I, Williams W, Webb G, et al. Pulmonary valve replacement late after repair of tetralogy of Fallot. *Ann Thorac Surg* 1997;64:526–530.

3. Ross J. Left ventricular function and the timing of surgical treatment in valvular heart disease. *Ann Intern Med* 1981;94:498–504.
4. Shimazaki V, Blackstone EH, Kirklin JW. The natural history of isolated congenital pulmonary valve incompetence: Surgical implications. *Thorac Cardiovasc Surg* 1984;32:257–259.
5. Gatzoulis MA, Till JA, Somerville J, et al. Mechano-electrical interaction in tetralogy of Fallot: QRS prolongation relates to right ventricular size and predicts malignant ventricular arrhythmias and sudden death. *Circulation* 1995;92:231–237.
6. Abd MY, Abdul-Khaliq H, Vogel M, et al. Relation between right ventricular enlargement, QRS duration, and right ventricular function in patients with tetralogy of Fallot and pulmonary regurgitation after surgical repair. *Heart* 2000;84:416–420.
7. Papavassiliou DP, Parks J, Hopkins KL, Fyfe DA. Three-dimensional echocardiographic measurement of right ventricular volume in children with congenital heart disease validated by magnetic resonance imaging. *J Am Soc Echocardiogr* 1998;11:770–777.
8. Goldberg SJ and Allen HD. Quantitative assessment by Doppler echocardiography of pulmonary or aortic regurgitation. *Am J Cardiol* 1985;56:131–135.
9. Eidem BW, O'Leary PW, Tei C, et al. Usefulness of the myocardial performance index for assessing right ventricular function in congenital heart disease. *Am J Cardiol* 2000;86:654–658.
10. Gatzoulis MA, Clark AL, Cullen S, et al. Right ventricular diastolic function 15–35 years after repair of tetralogy of Fallot. *Circulation* 1995;91:1775–1781.
11. Carvalho JS, Shinebourne EA, Busst C, et al. Exercise capacity after complete repair of tetralogy of Fallot: Deleterious effects of residual pulmonary regurgitation. *Brit Heart J* 1992;67:470–473.
12. Warner KG, Anderson JE, Fulton DR, et al. Restoration of pulmonary valve reduces right ventricular volume overload after previous repair of tetralogy of Fallot. *Circulation* 1993;88(Part 2):189–197.
13. Eyskens B, Reybrouck T, Bagaert J, et al. Homograft insertion for pulmonary regurgitation after repair of tetralogy of Fallot improves cardiorespiratory exercise performance. *Am J Cardiol* 2000;85:221–225.
14. Gatzoulis MA, Elliot JT, Guru V, et al. Right and left ventricular systolic function late after repair of tetralogy of Fallot. *Am J Cardiol* 2000;86:1352–1357.
15. Helbing WA, Rebergen MD, Maliepaard C, et al. Quantification of right ventricular function with magnetic resonance imaging in children with normal hearts and with congenital heart disease. *Am Heart J* 1995;130:828–837.
16. Lorenz CH, Walker EJ, Morgan VL, et al. Normal right and left ventricular mass systolic function, and gender differences by cine magnetic resonance imaging. *J Cardiovasc Mag Res* 1999;1:7–21.

Chapter V

Arrhythmia Management after Repair of Tetralogy of Fallot:

Preventing Sudden Death

J. Philip Saul, and
Andrew D. Blaufox

Introduction

A practical and academic problem in assessing risk factors for sudden cardiac death in patients following tetralogy repair is that these patients have an excellent overall survival rate. The studies that most effectively follow a cohort[1,2] identify only a total of 56 deaths out of 653 patients during a mean follow-up duration of 23 years. Of these deaths, 25% to 45% are identified as sudden cardiac death, while approximately one-third are the result of progressive myocardial failure. Even at the largest centers, this experience projects to only 1–3 serious events each year. So, how do we predict which patients are at risk, and how do we intervene?

Clinical Vignettes

The following vignettes represent actual events and data, but certain demographics have been altered in order to protect each patient's identity.

Case 1. A 30-year-old woman with tetralogy repaired with a transannular patch presented with palpitations and ventricular tachycardia (VT). After successful therapy with procainamide in the catheterization laboratory, she developed arthralgias and recurrent VT, prompting a referral.

Case 2. A 19-year-old man with tetralogy like double outlet right ventricle and pulmonary atresia, repaired with a two-stage procedure involving

From Gatzoulis MA, Murphy DJ (eds): *The Adult with Tetralogy of Fallot: The ISACCD Monograph Series* ©Futura Publishing Co., Inc, Armonk, NY, 2001.

ventricular septal defect closure and a right ventricular (RV) to pulmonary artery conduit at age 2, presented with sustained palpitations and near syncope, and a wide complex tachycardia at a rate of 270 beats/minute.

Case 3. A 17-year-old girl with complex tetralogy, who underwent a Rastelli procedure with ventricular septal defect closure to the aorta and RV to pulmonary artery conduit placement at age 4, and a conduit revision at age 17, presented 3 weeks after surgery with a brief episode of sustained palpitations and dizziness.

Case 4. A 26-year-old man with tetralogy repaired at age 6 following a systemic to pulmonary artery shunt presented with frequent asymptomatic non-sustained VT on Holter.

Case 5. A 19-year-old woman with tetralogy repaired at 8 months of age presented with acidosis and electro-mechanical dissociation after recieving brief cardiopulmonary resuscitation at the time of syncope. After recovery from further succesful resuscitation, electrocardiographic monitoring was unremarkable.

The Problem

Studies have shown overlap between hemodynamic, clinical, and electrocardiographic influences on VT and sudden death among patients who have undergone tetralogy repair.[3] Documented VT (Figure 1) or late sudden death occurs in late survivors of tetralogy, with one recent large study demonstrating a 6% incidence of sudden death at 30 years followup.[1] Numerous studies have now demonstrated a strong dependence of these outcomes on age at repair,[1] while other factors identified have been older age at follow-up,[4] RV pressure and/or volume overload,[1,3] a prior large systemic to pulmonary shunt,[5] a very wide QRS complex (>180 msec),[3] the presence of asymptomatic ventricular ectopy,[4] and the use of a transventricular versus a transatrial repair.[3] It should be noted that the issues of asymptomatic ectopy and the method of repair are somewhat controversial, since other studies have demonstrated no relation between sudden death and resting ventricular arrhythmias,[3] and numerous studies have found no relation between ventricular arrhythmias and the mild to moderate pulmonary regurgitation seen after transannular patch.[1] In addition, recent studies have demonstrated that a significant proportion of tetralogy patients have atrial tachycardias at late follow-up,[3,6] nearly a third in one study.[6] These atrial arrhythmias are another potential cause of sudden death in young patients with good atrioventricular (AV) node conduction and abnormal hemodynamics.[4] Importantly, the patients with atrial tachycardias may also have a high prevalence of ventricular arrhythmias on am-

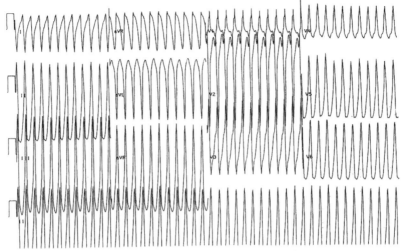

Figure 1. Twelve-lead electrocardiogram of patient 2 at presentation to a community hospital with palpitations, dyspnea and mildly decreased perfusion but without syncope. Of note is the rapid rate (273 bpm) with a wide QRS suggestive of LBBB and with evidence of VA dissociation.

bulatory monitoring,[3,6] leading to uncertainty about the etiology of events occurring in the absence of electrocardiographic monitoring.

Ventricular Tachycardia

The precise mechanism of sustained VT in patients with repaired tetralogy has been under some debate;[7] however, a variety of electrophysiological studies during induced tachycardia strongly support reentry as the likely mechanism.[8] Most of these investigators have assumed that the tachycardia circulates around the scar or patch in the RV outflow tract. That may be the case when there is no transannular patch, and the ventriculotomy does not extend to the pulmonary valve, leaving a conduction pathway circumferentially around the scar. However, detailed intraoperative mapping studies by Downer et al.[8] demonstrated endocardial macroreentry circuits that circulated around areas of functional rather than anatomic block in the RV outflow tract. Thus, reentrant circuits could be seen with transannular repairs, where a vertical ventriculotomy extends from at least the base of the infundibulum, across the pulmonary annulus and into the pulmonary artery, creating a line of complete conduction block at the superior margin of the infundibulum. These findings are also in agreement with the notion that microscopic fibrosis and myofiber dissarray in the RV outflow tract may be the basis of the late ventricular arrhythmias,[9] supporting the concept of early repair.

Electrophysiological Studies

As discussed above, the parameters reported for predicting which repaired patients are at risk for sustained VT or sudden death have either low sensitivity, as with the hemodynamic markers,[1,3] or low specificity and positive predictive value, as for the electrocardiographic markers.[3,4,10] Thus, one might hope that arrhythmia inducibility at electrophysiologic study could serve as more of a "gold standard", as it does for VT after myocardial infarction.[11] However, the existing data suggest that the problems of false positives and negatives seen after infarction[12] are only amplified in the tetralogy group.

At Children's Hospital, Boston, a study involving ventricular stimulation protocols in 140 patients with congenital heart disease, of whom 33% had undergone tetralogy repair, found only moderate predictive value for the electrophysiologic work-up of this disturbing problem.[13] The negative predictive value of a ventricular stimulation alone was 93%, the same as when patient characteristics, the occurrence of spontaneous VT, and the presence of symptoms were taken into consideration with each other. Reassurance against sudden cardiac death could be increased to 97% when a negative ventricular stimulation was considered with these other clinical variables. However, the positive predictive value of ventricular stimulation alone, although greater than any other clinical variable including spontaneous VT, was only 20%, which could only be raised to 24% when the stimulation results were combined with other clinical data. Despite the relatively low predictive value of a positive ventricular stimulation, when sustained, non-sustained and polymorphic VT were considered, a positive ventricular stimulation yielded a 6.1 times increased risk of all-cause mortality and a 3.2 times increased risk of sudden cardiac death. Furthermore, a positive ventricular stimulation predicted an approximately 40% all-cause mortality and an approximately 20% mortalitiy from sudden cardiac death at 8 years following stimulation, compared to 10% and 5% mortalities, respectively, for negative studies. When these and other results from intracardiac electrophysiologic evaluations[14] are combined with those from the electrocardiographic and hemodynamic evaluations discussed above, it is disturbingly clear that although malignant events are unlikely in patients with good hemodynamics, normal ambulatory monitoring and negative electrophysiological evaluations, no clinical parameters can be used to adequately rule out these events in many tetralogy patients.

Atrial Tachycardia

The role of atrial arrhythmias in producing postoperative morbidity and mortality is universally recognized after either an atrial switch repair for transposition of the great arteries[4] or the Fontan procedure for functional single ventricle;[15] however, the importance of atrial arrhythmias after other surgical repairs has not been equally emphasized, despite an often high prevalance.[6] As noted above, one recent study[6] found that 34% of repaired tetralogy patients had a history of atrial arrhythmias, with atrial flutter or fibrillation in 23% and "other" forms of supraventricular tachycardia in 11%, findings consistent with the outcome of Case #5 in this report (see below). Supraventricular tachycardia is particularly common in patients with severe symptoms, occurring in over 40% of our tetralogy patients with aborted sudden cardiac death or cardiac syncope (Figure 2).

Both animal and human electrophysiologic studies have established the reentrant nature of atrial tachycardias after cardiac surgery, and the importance of both anatomical and functional obstacles to atrial conduction in their initiation and maintenance.[16] The specific factors predisposing these patients to atrial reentry probably include 1) atrial scarring caused by multiple atriotomies, long suture lines and pericardial inflammation, 2) high atrial wall stress and hypertrophy due to increased pressure and chamber size,[3] 3) abnormal atrial anatomy associated with the underlying congenital lesion, and 4) changes in atrial refractoriness associated with sinus node dysfunction and concomitant bradycardia.[17]

In some of these patient groups, such as the atrial switch or Fontan patients, the atrial anatomy and electrophysiology are extremely complex, as

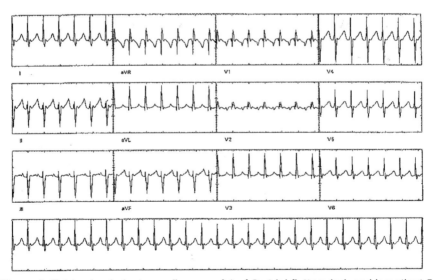

Figure 2. Twelve-lead electrocardiogram of 1 of 3 atrial flutters induced in patient 5. The atrial cycle length is 190 msec with 2:1 AV conduction. The expected baseline right bundle branch block, along with a superior axis counterclockwise loop suggestive of left anterior hemiblock.

reflected by the observation of multiple different tachycardia circuits.[18] In others, including the tetralogy and atrial septal defect (ASD) patients, the tachycardia may circulate around a single surgical or natural obstacle, such as an atriotomy scar, ASD patch, or the tricuspid valve.[19] Clearly, the electrophysiological complexity of the atrium will have a dramatic effect on the difficulty of therapies directed at altering the anatomic substrate of the arrhythmia, such as catheter ablation.

Summary—Pathophysiology

Patients with repaired tetralogy are at risk for sudden death. Although ventricular arrhythmias probably dominate the risk profile of these patients, atrial arrhythmias are also common and may play a role in the malignant events of some patients, particularly younger ones with minimal ventricular pathology, but excellent AV node conduction. Despite a myriad of associated influences, there is no set of clinical parameters, including the results of invasive electrophysiological testing, which can be used to adequately assess the risk of these events in individual patients.

Therapeutic Options

The goal of therapy in all patients with repaired tetralogy is clear—prevention of sudden death or severe hemodynamic compromise secondary to VT or a rapidly conducted atrial tachycardia. Although the ultimate therapy for achieving that goal, the internal cardioverter defibrillator (ICD), is now readily available, and comes in a package which allows for implantation with relatively low morbidity and close to zero mortality in adults and children,[20] it is probably not yet appropriate or feasible to implant such devices in all at risk patients. Thus, one is left with the options of no therapy, pharmacological antiarrhythmic prophylaxis, or directed catheter ablation in select patients. These therapeutic options will be discussed in a brief review of the available data below; however, as alluded to above, the dillema for these patients is probably as much what to do, than whom to do it to, a point which is well illustrated by the five cases outlined above. The management of these cases will be presented in detail after presentation of the options.

Antiarrhythmic Drug Therapy

Antiarrhythmic therapy directed by electrophysiological studies for inducible sustained monomorphic VT in patients with repaired tetralogy has the same limitations and advantages as in adults after myocardial infarction,[21] reasonable predictive value, but a significant risk of side effects, proarrhythmia and late drug failure, possibly due to evolution of the substrate.[8] However, the question of whether suppression of asymptomatic complex ventricular ectopy with drug therapy prevents sudden death in tetralogy patients has not yet been addressed in any prospective study, much less a large one similar to those available in adult patients after myocardial infarction.[21] Some investigators have strongly recommended suppressive therapy, primarily with dilantin,[4] on the basis of no sudden death after such therapy, while others have also found no sudden death in similar patients left unreated,[22] or treated only for symptoms.[23] Given these data and the known risk of malignant proarrhythmia with Class IA or C agents[24] and some Class III antiarrhythmic agents,[21] prophylactic therapy for asymptomatic patients with these agents probably makes little sense. Prophylaxis with more benign agents, such as dilantin or beta-blockade, is much less likely to be harmful; however, side effects are common with both therapies, and there is little firm data to support their use.

Internal Defibrillator Therapy

Since Mirowski et al.[25] first reported successful automatic internal defibrillation in humans, the ICD has had a dramatic impact on the management of and prognosis for adult patients at risk for sudden cardiac death, particularly for patients with good ventricular function, who are unlikely to die of non-arrhythmic causes.[26] Less data exist in pediatric patients. However, in a multicenter report of ICD use in 125 patients under 20 years of age, mortality was confined to the patients with abnormal ventricular function (9/46),[20] results very similar to those in adults. The 125 patients included 22 with congenital heart disease, 5 of whom had repaired tetralogy. Indications for implantation included aborted sudden cardiac death (76%), drug refractory VT (10%), unexplained syncope and induced arrhythmias (10%), and structural heart disease plus a family history of sudden death (4%). Appropriate ICD discharges occurred in 76% of the 60 patients followed for more than 24 months, and overall in 15 of the 22 patients with congenital heart disease (68%). Survival free from sudden cardiac death was 90% at 5 years for the entire group, and 95% for the patients with congenital heart disease.

Taken together, the adult and pediatric results suggest that ICD's can prevent sudden cardiac death in tetralogy patients with preserved left ventricular function. In addition, our own experience in 13 tetralogy patients has demonstrated adequate defibrillation thresholds (14.9 ± 6.9 J) using a transvenous approach, even in the presence of RV dilation secondary to pulmonary regurgitation. Initial survival analysis suggests a more favorable survival curve for patients treated with adjunctive ICD therapy, though follow-up is insufficient for confirmation of this hypothesis. Thus, the use of ICDs for secondary prevention is clearly supported in this patient population, and the rapid technological improvements in both the size and effectiveness of the devices suggest that primary prevention may be feasible in select patient groups. Unfortunately, the problem of selecting patients still remains. As more devices are placed, documentation of potentially life threatening arrhythmias will become available for analysis, thus allowing more precise identification of those who are truly at risk.

Catheter Ablation Therapy

Ventricular Tachycardia

There have now been a number of case reports and small series[27,28] describing successful ablation of VT in patients with tetralogy. This initial success supports the use of intracardiac ventricular stimulation in the algorithm for risk stratification, since patients with inducible VT may be offered ablative therapy. All successful ablations reported to date, and our own unreported ones (see Clinical Vignettes 1 and 4), have revealed a tachycardia mechanism consistent with macroreentry, and have involved RV tissue, either along the septum at the site of the ventricular septal defect repair, or in the anterior RV outflow tract (Figures 3 and 4). Although the anatomy is somewhat different, the potential for success is supported

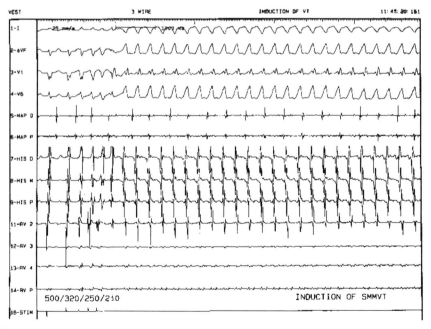

Figure 3. Induction of sustained ventricular tachycardia during programmed ventricular stimulation of patient 5.

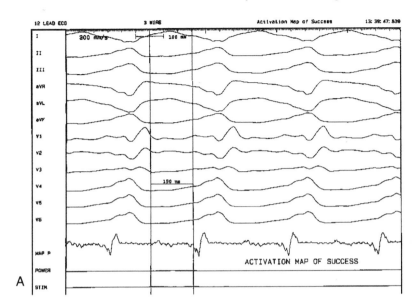

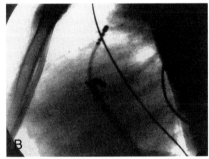

Figure 4. Electrograms from radiofrequency (RF) during RF catheter ablation of patient 5. Panel a: the activation map with fractionated potentials during early electrical diastole, 150 msec prior to the onset of the surface QRS or the earliest intracardiac ventricular electrograms. Panel b: Location of successful RF attempt. Panel c: RF application with ventricular tachycardia termination.

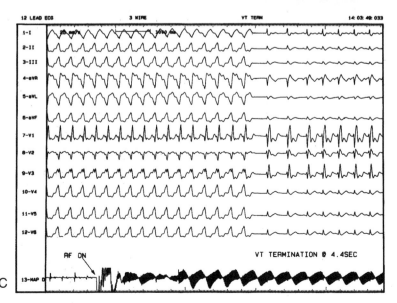

by the fact that the electrophysiologic substrate is similar to that found in macro-reentrant VTs following myocardial infarction, which are amenable to ablation, although less so than other VTs.[29] The recent development of electro-anatomic and non-contact mapping systems allows for better definition of underlying anatomy which may be beneficial in dealing with the added anatomic complexities of VT in repaired congenital heart disease. These systems have been shown to aid in the successful elimination of various VTs.[30] The ability to create a larger lesion with catheter tip cooling has led to larger lesion size and successful elimination of tachycardia without substantial differences in complications.[31] When such techniques are used in the postoperative anatomy in tetralogy, one might speculate that VT in this patient group may serve as the ideal model for catheter ablation of macroreentrant VT and outcomes will improve. Unfortunately, long-term follow-up demonstrating that new arrhythmia circuits do not arise post ablation is not yet available for any of these ablated patients.

Atrial Arrhythmias

The virtual failure of medical therapy to prevent recurrent atrial reentry tachycardia in patients with congenital heart disease[32] has lead to a natural interest in the use of radiofrequency (RF) catheter ablation techniques for this patient group. A few recent studies have reported the results of RF ablation for the treatment of atrial reentrant tachycardia in the setting of postoperative congenital heart disease.[18,33] While the success in all of these early studies has been achieved by targeting the "slow zone" of atrial conduction presumed necessary for maintenance of the reentry, some have emphasized the need for considering both the anatomy and electrophysiology simultaneously to identify a susceptible bridge of tissue with the correct properties.[18,33] Such an approach requires careful review of the details of atrial surgery, in addition to detailed mapping of the reentry circuit, using entrainment pacing similar to that used for post-infarction VT in adults.[34] Using such an approach at Children's Hospital, Boston, successful tachycardia interruption was achieved in 8 of the first 10 patients (80%), and 17 of 22 atrial reentry circuits (77%), at a wide diversity of anatomic locations.[18] The availability of electrophysiology catheters with a high density of electrodes capable of simultaneously mapping the entire atria may facilitate rapid identification of multiple reentry circuits and increase the initial success rate.[35] The more recent advances in tachycardia mapping using electro-anatomic magnetic or non-contact technologies have also been applied to atrial arrhythmias.[36,37] Not only do these systems allow for identification of circuit location[36] and anatomic definition (Figure 5), they also allow for easy assessment of post-ablation conduction block[38,39] which improves success.[40] In South Carolina, our early experience, during 1998 and 1999, has yielded a success rate of 91% in 34 cases, 6 performed with electroanatomic mapping and 28 with traditional entrainment methods alone. The elec-

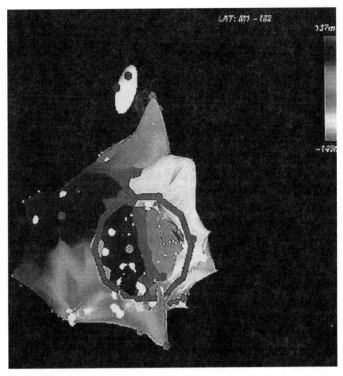

Figure 5. Atypical clockwise flutter is depicted by electroanatomic magnetic mapping which demonstrates that the circuit involves "a peri-valvar pouch" just inferior and lateral to the tricuspid valve annulus. The circuit was eliminated with a series of lesions in this isthmus area including this pouch. This anatomic detail is not seen in traditional fluoroscopy.

troanatomic system also allows for assessment and prophylactic block of other potential circuits not necessarily induced during the study,[37] thus potentially decreasing recurrence rates. No data currently exist to support or refute this hypothesis. However when advanced mapping technologies are combined with cooled tip technology, the potential for long-term cure is hopeful. The natural history of atrial arrhythmia recurrence in this patient population suggests that long-term follow-up will be necessary well before declaring victory. Fortunately, as noted above, the reentry circuit in patients with less complex atrial anatomy, such as that seen in tetralogy, is more likely to be single, enhancing the chance of successful ablation.[19]

Hemodynamic/Arrhythmia Surgery

Hemodynamic factors, such as valvar incompetence[3] and residual outflow obstruction which lead to pressure and volume overload[1,3] are associated with arrhythmias and sudden death. Thus, relief of these hemodynamic residua may lead to lower incidences of arrhythmia and sudden death. Unfortunately, the data concerning this approach to management is sparse and incomplete. While the limited data available does suggest improvement in symptoms of right heart failure[41,42] and good intermediate survival,[41,42] no reduction in the risk of sudden death has been shown.[41–43] However, there may be some decrease in arrhythmias, if antiarrhythmic cryoablation is performed concurrently.[42] Although the abolishment of arrhythmias has not been shown to diminish sudden cardiac death in these patients,[41,42] the number of patients have been small and the duration of follow up has been short.

Perhaps more challenging than the decision to recommend surgical reintervention, is the decision *when* to have it done. In a recent study involving patients who underwent late primary tetralogy repair, and who underwent reintervention approximately 20 years later, the ability to improve hemodynamics was limited in the subgroup with RV ejection fractions below 40% despite improvement of symptoms.[43] While differences in arrhythmia and sudden cardiac death incidences were not measured, one is left with the impression that there may be a point at which surgical reintervention alone will be insufficient to prevent arrhythmia and sudden cardiac death.

Clinical Vignettes

Case 1. After referral, initial evaluation of the 30-year-old woman with tetralogy and VT began with an echocardiogram, which revealed a dilated right ventricle due to free pulmonary regurgitation. She underwent cardiac catheterization with a hemodynamic and electrophysiological evaluation. Except for the dilated right ventricle, there were excellent post tetralogy repair hemodynamics without residual shunts. Sustained VT identical to her clinical tachycardia could be induced with 3 ventricular extrastimuli (Figure 3). Application of RF energy was applied in the RV outflow tract, resulting in tachycardia termination and noninducibility (Figure 4). Tachycardia was also not inducible at a follow-up electrophysiological evaluation 6 weeks later.

Case 2. The 19-year-old young man with tetralogy, sustained palpitations, near-syncope and rapid monomorphic VT (Figure 1) underwent catheterization which revealed RV outflow tract obstruction resulting in near systemic pressure in the right ventricle, mildy elevated left ventricular filling pressure, reduced cardiac output, and elevated pulmonary vascular resistance. An electrophysiological evaluation revealed normal sinus and AV node function, and non-sustained atrial reentry with rapid atrial pacing; however, aggressive ventricular stimulation performed at 4 sites (3 right ventricle and 1 left ventricle), and with isoproterenol at 2 sites never produced sustained VT. Consequently, he underwent two surgical procedures for conduit revision and placement of a transvenous ICD. Over the subsequent 6 months, he had 6 appropriate ICD discharges to successfully terminate VT at rates of 280–290 beats/minute (Figure 6), despite initial negative ventricular stimulation. Repeat programmed stimulation using the ICD and on isoproterenol finally induced VT at a rate of just over 300 beats/minute. Ablation therapy was considered, but deferred due to limited venous access, pending a clinical trial of amiodarone to reduce the number of shocking events.

Case 3. Following her initial syncopal episode, this 17-year-old was monitored during a multiple day admission. Only rare atrial and ventricular premature beats were seen on bedside and Holter monitoring, and an echocardiogram revealed minimal RV outflow tract obstruction and good left ventricular function. Non-sustained atrial flutter was induced at an esophageal electrophysiological study, and was felt to be consistent with her symptoms and early postoperative status. She was placed on digoxin and discharged, but 2 weeks later had recurrent palpitations without dizziness, and

Onset VT
290 bpm

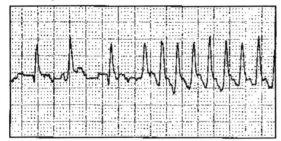

Therapy Delivered
10 J. Biphasic

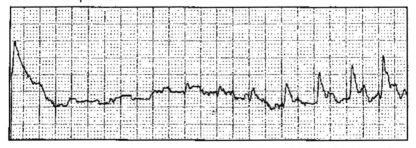

Figure 6. The top panel demonstrates the onset of a rapid clinical tachycardia, with a rate of 295 bpm in patient 2. A successful shock from an ICD converted him to sinus rhythm.

was readmitted. An intracardiac electrophysiology study revealed normal sinus and AV node function, again non-sustained atrial flutter, and no inducible ventricular arrhythmias with up to 3 extrastimuli at a single site, without isoproterenol. She was given beta-blockade and discharged with an event monitor and a presumed diagnosis of atrial flutter. She died suddenly on the bus to school 11 days later after activating the event monitor (Figure 7).

Case 4. The asymptomatic 26-year-old man with non-sustained VT had a QRS duration of 190 msec on surface electrocardiogram. A catheterization revealed excellent hemodynamics. An electrophysiological evaluation revealed non-sustained atrial reentry with single atrial premature beats, but sustained reproducible monomorphic VT at a rate of 200 beats/minute using an S3 protocol. He remained asymptomatic on mexilitine, but 2 years later the mexilitene was discontinued and he underwent successful RF ablation of a single VT circuit in the RV outflow tract (Figure 8).

Case 5. Although standard resuscitative efforts and medications led to a prompt hemodynamic recovery in the 19-year-old woman with syncope, relatively severe ischemic brain injury had been sustained during the event. Initial echocardiographic evaluation revealed minimal RV outflow

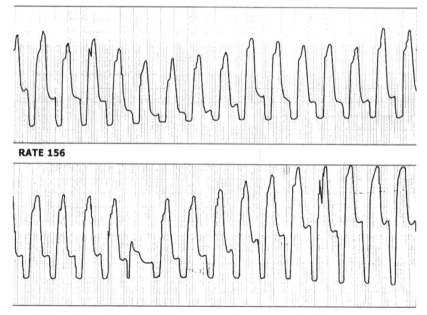

RATE 156

Figure 7. A portion of the third of four pages of a memory looping event monitor triggered by patient 3 during a fatal episode of sustained ventricular tachycardia (VT). In the bottom panel, a sinus fusion beat confirms the clinical diagnoses of VT.

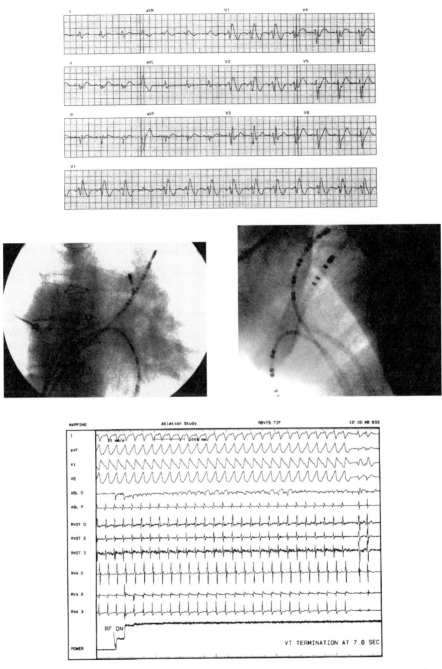

Figure 8. Location and termination of sustained ventricular tachycardia VT in patient 4 during successful radiofrequency catheter ablation of his VT. This patient had high grade ectopy and no significant symptoms, but reproducible VT on repeated electrophysiologic studies.

tract obstruction, mild to moderate pulmonary regurgitation, and mildly depressed left ventricular function. Although ventricular ectopy was present during the first 48 hours, sinus tachycardia was the only arrhythmia seen during 4 weeks of subsequent observation. Catheterization 3 weeks after the event revealed excellent hemodynamics with a minimal RV outflow tract gradient, no inducible ventricular arrhythmias with an S4 protocol in 2 sites with 2 cycle lengths and 1 site with isoproterenol. Atrial stimulation easily induced sustained typical atrial flutter[44] which appeared to proceed counterclockwise around the tricuspid valve (Figure 2). The atrial flutter was terminated and conduction block in the tricuspid-inferior vena cava isthmus produced using linear applications of RF energy between the tricspid annulus and inferior vena cava.[45] No arrythmias could be induced post ablation. She was discharged to long-term rehabilitation on digoxin and atenolol. Atrial flutter was noninducible at a follow-up atrial stimulation study performed 4 months after the ablation, and no arryhthmias were observed during a year of follow-up.

Summary

These six cases demonstrate a number of important issues concerning the assessement and reduction of sudden cardiac death risk in tetralogy patients. First, and perhaps foremost, there are no clinical parameters which can be used to accurately assess the risk. Although poor hemodynamics and ventricular ectopy on ambulatory monitoring are reasonably sensitive indicators,[46] they still fail to identify many patients at high risk, such as the two patients of Cases 3 and 5. Second, the data from intracardiac electrophysiological evaluations may be even worse at identifying the at-risk population, as demonstrated by Cases 2 and 3, and by the multicenter Pediatric Electrophysiology Society experience.[47] In addition, as shown in Case 4, the low specificity of electrophysiological studies in this patient group[48] leaves even the interpretation of inducible monorphic VT in question, although it is clear that such findings are hard to ignore. Third, pharmacological agents which appear to be successful by inducibility criteria may fail as chronic therapy, as occurred in Case 1. Fourth, catheter ablation can be acutely successful, eliminating the short-term need for antiarrhythmic drug therapy and its side effects (Cases 1 and 4), but the long term efficacy of ablation in preventing recurrent VT is unknown. Fifth, aborted sudden cardiac death in tetralogy patients may not always be due to VT, requiring a thorough investigation for atrial arrhythmias even in those patients with complex ventricular ectopy on ambulatory electrocardiographic monitoring. Sixth, coexistent hemodynamic issues need to be sought and corrected. However, data on arrhythmia benefit from surgical intervention and restoration of haemodynamics are limited at present. Finally, it is clear that no single evaluation or therapy can be used for assessing the risk of or preventing sudden cardiac death in patients who have undergone surgery for tetralogy.

Controversies/Unresolved Issues

Based on the data and cases presented above, it is clear that there are a number issues which require additional data for their ultimate resolution. First and foremost is the identification of the patient at risk for potentially malignant ventricular arrhythmias. Both past and more recent data[10,49] have drawn attention to some of these risk factors, but no combination lowers false negative and false positive outcomes enough to have acceptable sensitivity and specificity. Next, once the at-risk patient is finally identified, the optimum management remains unclear, with the possible exception that drug therapy remains an inadequate choice. Although one would like to rely on successful catheter ablation as a long-term cure, there is currently no data to support such a contention, such that most patients probably deserve a follow-up ventricular stimulation study at some point more than 1 month after the procedure. Devices remain another option, either with or without ablation. However, despite vast improvements in ICD technology, given the low sudden death rates in even the at risk population[2] and the potential risks of ICDs,[50] primary prevention with ICD placement in the absence of symptoms may not yet be the solution. Further, ICDs may succeed in converting patients to a more stable rhythm, but they cannot correct associated electromechanical dissociation. Finally, all of the diagnostic and therapeutic management issues discussed above for ventricular arrhythmias apply to atrial reentrant arrhythmias as well, further complicating the overall management of these patients. Dr. Amnon Rosenthal may have summarized the issues involved in the management of postoperative tetralogy patients best with the title of his 1993 editorial:[51] "Adults with tetralogy of Fallot—repaired yes: cured, no." Clearly, there is much work to be done.

References

1. Murphy JG, Gersh BJ, Mair DD, et al. Long-term outcome in patients undergoing surgical repair of tetralogy of Fallot. *New Engl J Med* 1993;329:593–599.
2. Nollert G, Fischlein T, Bouterwet S, et al. Long-term survival in patients with repair of Tetralogy of Fallot: 36-year follow-up of 490 survivors of the first year after surgical repair. *JACC* 1997;30:1374–1383.
3. Gatzoulis MA, Balaji S, Webber S, et al. Risk factors for arrhythmia and sudden cardiac death late after repair of tetralogy of Fallot: A multicentre study. *Lancet* 2000;356:975–981.
4. Garson A Jr., Randall DC, Gillette PC, et al. Prevention of sudden death after repair of tetralogy of Fallot: Treatment of ventricular arrhythmias. *JACC* 1985;6:221–227.

5. Katz NM, Blackstone EH, Kirklin JW, et al. Late survival and symptoms after repair of tetralogy of Fallot. *Circulation* 1982;65:403–410.
6. Roos-Hesselink J, Perlroth MG, McGhie J, et al. Atrial arrhythmias in adults after repair of tetralogy of Fallot. Correlations with clinical, exercise, and echocardiographic findings. *Circulation* 1995;91:2214–2219.
7. Garson A, Jr. Ventricular dysrhythmias after congenital heart surgery: A canine model. *Pediatric Research* 1984;18:1112–1120.
8. Downar E, Harris L, Kimber S, et al. Ventricular tachycardia after surgical repair of tetralogy of Fallot: Results of intraoperative mapping studies. *JACC* 1992;20:648–655.
9. Kawai S, Okada R, Kitamura K, et al. A morphometrical study of myocardial disarray associated with right ventricular outflow tract obstruction. *Japanese Circulation Journal* 1984;48:445–456.
10. Gatzoulis MA, Till JA, Somerville J, et al. Mechano-electrical interaction in tetralogy of Fallot: QRS prolongation relates to right ventricular size and predicts malignant ventricular arrhythmias and sudden death. *Circulation* 1995; 92:231–237.
11. Wellens HJ, Brugada P, Stevenson WG. Programmed electrical stimulation of the heart in patients with life-threatening ventricular arrhythmias: What is the significance of induced arrhythmias and what is the correct stimulation protocol? *Circulation* 1985;72:1–7.
12. Trappe HJ, Brugada P, Talajic M, et al. Value of induction of pleomorphic ventricular tachycardia during programmed stimulation. *Eur Heart J* 1989; 10:133–141.
13. Alexander ME, Walsh EP, Saul JP, et al. Value of programmed ventricular stimulation in patients with congenital heart disease. *J Cardiovasc Electrophysiol* 1999;10:1033–1044.
14. Deal BJ, Scagliotti D, Miller SM, et al. Electrophysiologic drug testing in symptomatic ventricular arrhythmias after repair of tetralogy of Fallot. *Am J Cardiol* 1987;59:1380–1385.
15. Fishberger SB, Wernovsky G, Gentles TL, et al. Factors that influence the development of atrial flutter after the fontan operation. *J Thorac Cardiovasc Surg* 1997;113:80–86.
16. Gillette PC, Kugler JD, Garson A Jr., et al. Mechanisms of cardiac arrhythmias after the Mustard operation for transposition of the great arteries. *Am J Cardiol* 1980; 45:1225–1230.
17. Flinn CH, Wolff GS, Dick II M. Cardiac rhythm after the Mustard operation for complete transposition of the great arteries. *N Engl J Med* 1984;310:1635–1638.
18. Triedman JK, Saul JP, Weindling SN, et al. Radiofrequency ablation of intra-atrial reentrant tachycardia after surgical palliation of congenital heart disease. *Circulation* 1995;91:707–714.
19. Kalman JM, VanHare GF, Olgin JE, et al. Ablation of "incisional" reentrant atrial tachycardia complicating surgery for congenital heart disease: Use of entrainment to define a critical isthmus of conduction. *Circulation* 1996; 93:502–512.
20. Silka MJ, Kron J, Dunnigan A, et al. Sudden cardiac death and the use of implantable cardioverter- defibrillators in pediatric patients. The Pediatric Electrophysiology Society. *Circulation* 1993;87:800–807.
21. Waldo AL, Camm AJ, deRuyter H, et al. Effect of d-sotalol on mortality in patients with left ventricular dysfunction after recent and remote myocardial infarction. The SWORD Investigators. Survival With Oral d-Sotalol. *Lancet* 1996;348:7–12.
22. Cullen S, Celermajer DS, Franklin RC, et al. Prognostic significance of ventric-

ular arrhythmia after repair of tetralogy of Fallot: A 12-year prospective study. *JACC* 1994;23:1151–1155.

23. Vaksmann G, Fournier A, Davignon A, et al. Frequency and prognosis of arrhythmias after operative "correction" of tetralogy of Fallot. *Am J Cardiol* 1990;66:346–349.

24. Echt DS, Liebson PR, Mitchell LB, et al. Mortality and morbidity in patients receiving encainide, flecainide, or placebo. The Cardiac Arrhythmia Suppression Trial. *N Engl J Med* 1991:324;781–788.

25. Mirowski M, Reid PR, Mower MM, et al. Termination of malignant ventricular arrhythmias with an implanted automatic defibrillator in human beings. *N Engl J Med* 1980;303:322–324.

26. Zipes DP, DiMarco JP, Gillette PC, et al. Guidelines for clinical intracardiac electrophysiological and catheter ablation procedures. A report of the American College of Cardiology/American Heart Association Task Force on Practice Guidelines (Committee on Clinical Intracardiac Electrophysiologic and Catheter Ablation Procedures), developed in collaboration with the North American Society of Pacing and Electrophysiology. *JACC* 1995;26:555–573.

27. Biblo LA, Carlson MD. Transcatheter radiofrequency ablation of ventricular tachycardia following surgical correction of tetralogy of Fallot. *PACE* 1994; 17:1556–1560.

28. Chinushi M, Aizawa Y, Kitazawa H, et al. Clockwise and counter-clockwise circulation of wavefronts around an anatomical obstacle as one mechanism of two morphologies of sustained ventricular tachycardia in patients after a corrective operation of tetrology of Fallot. *PACE* 1997;20:2279–2281.

29. Scheinman MM, Huang S. The1998 NASPE prospective catheter ablation registry. *PACE* 2000;23,1020–1028.

30. Friedman PA, Beinborn DA, Schultz J, et al. Ablation of noninducible idiopathic left ventricular tachycardia using a noncontact map acquired from a premature complex with tachycardia morphology. *PACE* 2000;23:1311–1314.

31. Calkins H, Epstein AE, Packer D, et al. Catheter ablation of ventricular tachycardia in patients with structural heart disease using cooled radiofrequency energy: Results of a prospective multicenter study. Cooled RF Multicenter Investigational Group. *JACC* 2000;35:1905–1914.

32. Weindling SN, Saul JP, Triedman JK, et al. Recurrent intra-atrial reentry tachycardia following congential heart disease surgery: The search for an optimum therapy. *Circulation* 1995;92:I-765 Abstract.

33. Lesh MD, Van Hare GF, Epstein LM, et al. Radiofrequency catheter ablation of atrial arrhythmias. Results and mechanisms. *Circulation* 1994;89:1074–1089.

34. Stevenson WG, Khan H, Sager P, et al. Identification of reentry circuit sites during catheter mapping and radiofrequency ablation of ventricular tachycardia late after myocardial infarction. *Circulation* 1993;88(Pt 1):1647–1670.

35. Triedman JK, Bergau DM, Saul JP, et al. Efficacy of radiofrequency ablation for control of intraatrial rentrant tachcyardia in patients with congenital heart disease. *JACC* 1997;30:1032–1038.

36. Collins KK, Love BA, Walsh E, et al. Location of acutely successful radiofrequency ablation of intraatrial reentrant tachycardia in patients with congenital heart disease. *Am J Cardiol* 2000;86:969–974.

37. Love BA, Collins KK, Walsh EP, et al. Conduction corridors for intraatrial reentrant tachycardia in congenital heart disease are predicted by electroanatomic mapping during sinus/paced rhythm. *Circulation* 1999:100; I-803.

38. Sra J, Bhatia A, Dhala A, et al. Electroanatomic mapping to identify breakthrough sites in recurrent typical human flutter. *PACE* 2000;23:1479–1492.

39. Coyne RF, Deely M, Gottlieb CD, et al. Electroanatomic Magnetic Mapping dur-

ing Ablation of Isthmus-dependent Atrial Flutter. *J Interv Card Electrophysiol* 2000;4:635–643.

40. Kottkamp H, Hugl B, Krauss B, et al. Electromagnetic versus fluoroscopic mapping of the inferior isthmus for ablation of typical atrial flutter: A prospective randomized study. *Circulation* 2000;102:2082–2086.

41. Yemets IM, Williams WG, Webb GD, et al. Pulmonary valve replacement late after repair of tetralogy of Fallot. *Ann Thorac Surg* 1997;64:526–530.

42. Oechslin EN, Harrison DA, Harris L, et al. Reoperation in adults with repair of tetralogy of fallot: Indications and outcomes. *J Thorac Cardiovasc Surg* 1999;118;245–251.

43. Therrien J, Siu S, McLaughlin PR, et al. Pulmonary valve replacement in adults late after repair of tetralogy of Fallot: Are we operating too late? *J Am Coll Cardiol* 2000;36:1670–1675.

44. Saxon LA, Kalman JM, Olgin JE, et al. Results of radiofrequency catheter ablation for atrial flutter. *Am J Cardiol* 1996;77:1014–1016.

45. Nakagawa H, Lazzara R, Khastgir T, et al. Role of the tricuspid annulus and the eustachian valve/ridge on atrial flutter. Relevance to catheter ablation of the septal isthmus and a new technique for rapid identification of ablation success [see comments]. *Circulation* 1996;94:407–424.

46. Garson A, Jr. Ventricular arrhythmias after repair of congenital heart disease: Who needs treatment? *Cardiology in the Young* 1991;1:177–181.

47. Chandar JS, Wolff GS, Garson A Jr., et al. Ventricular arrhythmias in postoperative tetralogy of Fallot. *Am J Cardiol* 1990;65:655–661.

48. Balaji S, Lau YR, Case CL, et al. QRS prolongation is associated with inducible ventricular tachycardia after repair of tetralogy of Fallot. *Am J Cardiol* 1997;80:160–163.

49. Gatzoulis MA, Till JA, Redington AN. Depolarization-repolarization inhomogeneity after repair of tetralogy of Fallot. The substrate for malignant ventricular tachycardia? *Circulation* 1997;95:401–404.

50. Gold MR, Peters RW, Johnson JW, et al. Complications associated with pectoral cardioverter- defibrillator implantation: Comparison of subcutaneous and submuscular approaches. Worldwide Jewel Investigators. *JACC* 1996;28:1278–1282.

51. Rosenthal A. Adults with tetralogy of Fallot—repaired, yes; cured no. *N Engl J Med* 1993;329:655–656

Chapter VI

Reoperation Late after Repair of Tetralogy of Fallot: Indication, Timing and, Outcome

William G. Williams, Louise Harris,
Eugene Downer, Glen S.VanArsdell,
Peter R. McLaughlin, and Gary D.Webb

Introduction

Lillihei first reported surgical repair of tetralogy of Fallot in 1955. Long-term survival of patients from that sentinel experience is surprisingly good.[1] However, late complications after repair of tetralogy in childhood became widely recognized; an increasing prevalence of right heart failure, arrhythmia and sudden death,[2–5] and less commonly, left heart problems. Castaneda proposed that early repair during infancy, and avoiding palliative operations, would improve both early and late results.[6] He pioneered successful techniques for primary repair in neonates and infants in the 1970s that established the standard for management of infants with tetralogy in the present era.

It is increasingly uncommon for patients with unrepaired tetralogy to present as adults. Conversely, due to the success of improving care during childhood, there is an almost exponential increase in the number of adults with previous repair of tetralogy. Some of these adults may require reoperation. Most adults underwent repair at a much older age, and with a greater likelihood of palliative operations prior to repair than is common practice in the current era. As Deanfield has written, "Long follow-up inevitably means surgery in an earlier era: More recent surgery, at a younger

From Gatzoulis MA, Murphy DJ (eds): *The Adult with Tetralogy of Fallot: The ISACCD Monograph Series* ©Futura Publishing Co., Inc., Armonk, NY, 2001.

age, with better preoperative, operative, and post-operative care will improve long-term results."[7]

We report our experience with surgical management of adults with tetralogy requiring reoperation late after previous repair within the context of these evolving trends.

Methods

The computerized database of the surgical division was searched for all operations for adults with tetralogy from 1972 to December 31, 2000. One hundred and eleven patients were identified. Fifty-four patients who were first repaired as adults were excluded from this analysis, except for 4 who required a reoperation late after repair. Clinic files, office records & notes from referring physicians were reviewed for a cross-sectional follow-up extending to 1999 or 2000.

Prevalence

Tetralogy of Fallot accounts for about 10% of all forms of congenital heart disease among infants and children.[8] Its prevalence in adults is less certain. "Adult" is defined in our health care system as an admission to the Toronto General Hospital, generally older than age 18 years. To date, of the 111 adults who have had late reoperation after tetralogy repair, 65 were referred from our own clinic. Our adult congenital cardiac clinic follows 5,745 patients (years 1982 to 2000), among whom there are 500 patients with repaired tetralogy. Therefore the *surgical* patients who underwent reoperation represent 1.6% of the total clinic population, and 13% of the tetralogy clinic patients. Further, we estimate that of the childhood repairs of tetralogy at the adjacent Hospital for Sick Children, 1,500 are now older than age 18 years. Consequently, the locally referred 65 adult surgical patients having a late reoperation represent 4.3% of the tetralogy population who are presently older than age 18 years.

The total population of adult congenital patients having *surgery* by our group is 1,282, therefore the 111 reoperation tetralogy patients comprise 8.7% of all our congenital cardiac surgical patients.

Reoperation in Adults Late after tetralogy Repair

Reoperation late after repair of tetralogy was performed in 111 adults. Four have required a subsequent reoperation, therefore the total number of reoperations is 115. The age at reoperation is a median of 35.6 years (range 16.5–62.3 years) (Figure 1). The interval from initial repair to late reoperation is a median of 23.6 years (range 6–39.3 years). Most of these patients had their repair during childhood, but 17 were over age 18 years

Age at Initial Repair

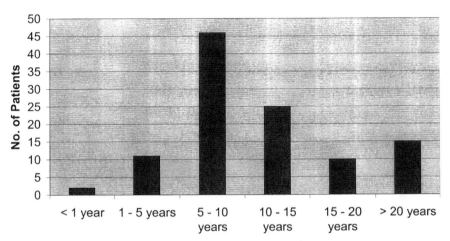

Figure 1. Age at initial repair among 111 adults requiring reoperation. Median age is 9.5 years (range 0.3–56 years). Seventeen patients were older than age 18 years at initial repair.

prior to initial repair, including four repaired by our group. Mean age at repair was 9.4 years (mean 12.4, range 0.3–56 years). Palliative operations prior to repair, were used in 44% of these patients. Fifty-one percent had a transannular patch repair and all were repaired through a right ventriculotomy.

The number of reoperations each year is increasing, as illustrated (Figure 2).

The primary indications for reoperation are right ventricular outflow tract lesions, (81% of the reoperations), and arrhythmia (Table 1).

Right ventricular outflow tract lesions are pulmonary valve insufficiency (54 patients, 48% of the total), and less commonly, stenosis (27 patients) or both (6 patients). Among patients with stenosis, 16 had stenosis in a previous pulmonary conduit, 5 in the native valve, 4 at infundibular level, and 2 at the branch pulmonary arteries. Branch pulmonary artery stenosis was present in 44 patients as a secondary lesion.

Most patients (74%) had one or more associated lesions (Table 2).

Arrhythmia, although not common as the primary indication for reoperation (n=3), was present in 47 patients (43%) prior to reoperation. Ventricular tachycardia (VT) was present in 24 patients, supraventricular in 16, and both in 5. There were also 2 patients with intermittent sinus arrest. In all patients with VT or supraventricular tachycardia, intraoperative electrophysiologic mapping was carried out as previously described.[9] Those patients who could be mapped and had unifocal VT underwent

Late Re-operation after Tetralogy Repair

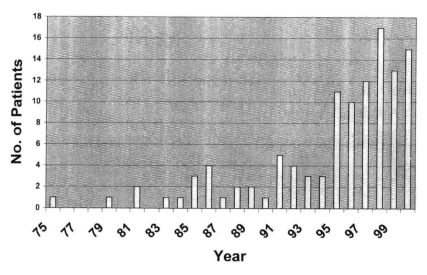

Figure 2. Adult tetralogy reoperations by year of operation. Seventy percent of reoperations occurred after 1994. Mean age at reoperation is 35 years, (range 16.5–56 years), and at initial repair, 9.5 years.

cryothermic ablation. For atrial flutter, cryoablation of the inferior vena cava-to-right atrial junction to the atrial septum was performed, and for those with atrial flutter and fibrillation, a modified right atrial maze operation was used.[10]

Table 1.
Primary Diagnosis in 111 Late Reoperations.

	N
Pulmonary Insufficiency	54
Prosthetic Pulmonary valve failure	16
Pulmonary Stenosis	5
Pulmonary Stenosis & Insufficiency	6
Right ventricular outflow obstruction	4
Pulmonary artery Branch stenosis	2
Patent shunt	3
Ventricular septal defect	8
Tricuspid Insufficiency	6
Arrhythmia	3
Aortic Insufficiency	3
Left ventricular aneurysm	1
	111

Table 2.
Associated Diagnosis.

	N
Tricuspid insufficiency	22
Pulmonary artery Branch Stenosis	16
Right ventricular outflow Aneurysm	15
Atrial septal defect	8
Ventricular septal defect	8
Pulmonary stenosis	8
Pulmonary insufficiency	7
Absent Pulmonary valve syndrome	4
Aortic insufficiency	1
Aortic Aneurysm	1
Coronary from pulmonary artery	1
Aortic coarctation	1
Subaortic stenosis	1
Coronary artery stenosis	1
	94

Results

Reoperation in Adults Late After Tetralogy Repair

An orthotopically positioned pulmonary valve tissue prosthesis was implanted in 90 patients (83%). Concomitant procedures were required in all but 6 patients. Arrhythmia ablation was performed in 39 patients (35% of the total). The other surgical procedures are listed in Tables 3 and 4.

There was one early death (vide infra).

During follow-up (median 4.4 years, range 0–24 years), five late deaths have occurred. The late deaths occurred between 0.7–8.8 years (median 7.7 years) post reoperation, at ages 37–73 years (median 61). The indica-

Table 3.
Surgical Procedures at Reoperation.

Pulmonary valve Implant	90
Arrhythmia Ablation	39
Pulmonary artery Arterioplasty	46
Tricuspid valve Repair	24
Right ventricular outflow resection	22
Right ventricular "Aneurysm"	22
Atrial septal defect	20
Ventricular septal defect	14
Subaortic resection	1
Total Procedures	278

Table 4.
Reoperation Late after Tetralogy Repair.

Primary Procedure at Reoperation

	N
Pulmonary valve implantation	83
Ventricular septal defect	7
Aortic valve replacement	3
Arrhythmia	3
Tricuspid valve repair/replace	6
Right ventricular outflow resection	4
Pulmonary artery plasty/shunt takedown	4
Left ventricular aneurysm	1
Total patients	111

tions for reoperation among these 5 were a residual ventricular septal defect in 2, pulmonary stenosis in 1, and pulmonary regurgitation in 1, each had a pulmonary valve implantation, and tricuspid regurgitation requiring replacement in a patient with persistent supraventricular tachycardia & right heart failure. The cause of death was congestive heart failure in the 2 oldest patients, sudden in 1 (no arrhythmia prior to reoperation) and unknown in 2. Survival by Kaplan Meier analysis is 84% ± 8% at 10 years after reoperation (Figure 3).

There are, to date, four further reoperations among the 110 operative

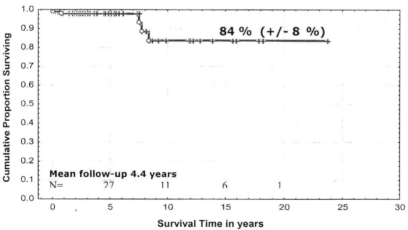

Figure 3. Survival analysis of 111 adults undergoing reoperation late after tetralogy repair.

survivors. The initial reoperation was for VT in 1, pulmonary valve insufficiency in 2, and aortic insufficiency in 1. The indication for subsequent reoperation was pulmonary regurgitation with VT in 1, pulmonary stenosis in the 2 patients with pulmonary regurgitation, one of whom also had VT, and aortic regurgitation with aortic root aneurysm requiring a Bentall operation. Kaplan Meier analysis for survival free of reoperation or death at 5, 10, and 15 years is 95%, 77%, and 62% respectively (Figure 4).

Arrhythmia ablation was performed in 39 of the 47 patients with preoperative arrhythmia. Ablation could not be performed in patients with multifocal VT, or those in whom the arrhythmia could not be elicited during surgery and electrophysiologic mapping. The most common site of the VT re-entry circuit was the superior margin of the ventricular septal defect suture line, i.e., the infundibular septum and its parietal extension. Cryoablation to interrupt the VT pathway was performed in 19 of the 24 patients with VT.

Fifteen of the 16 patients with supraventricular tachycardia underwent a cryoablation of the inferior vena cava right atrial junction or a right atrial maze procedure. All five patients with both VT & supraventricular tachycardia had a combined cryoablation of infundibular septum and the inferior vena cava right atrial junction.

Among the 39 with ablation, one early death occurred, a 43-year-old man with supraventricular tachycardia and hypoplastic pulmonary arter-

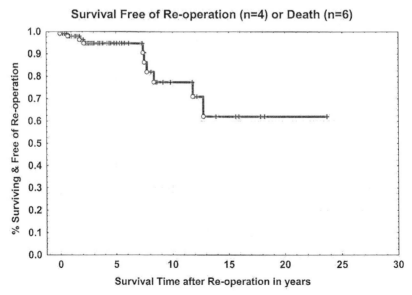

Figure 4. Survival free of either death or reoperation. At 10 years after surgery, 76% of patients are free of either complication.

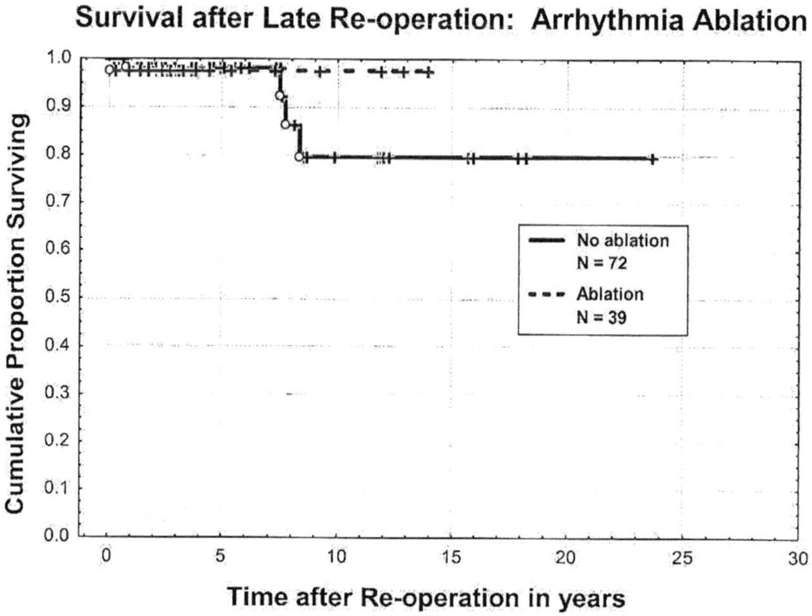

Survival after Late Re-operation: Arrhythmia Ablation

Figure 5. Survival after reoperation among patients with ablation of arrhythmia (n = 39) compared to 72 patients who did not have ablation. There is 1 death among the ablation patients and 4 among the others. There is no statistically significant difference in survival.

ies. Death was due to low cardiac output after bilateral pulmonary arterioplasty and replacement of the pulmonary valve and ascending aorta.

Long-term survival among patients with cryoablation is at least comparable to those without preoperative arrhythmia (Figure 5). There are no deaths in the 8 with arrhythmia who did not have ablation, 6 of whom had VT, and 2, sinus arrest. During follow-up, among the patients treated for VT, 2 underwent a subsequent reoperation for VT, and 1 had placement of an ICD.

Discussion

Current management of patients with tetralogy of Fallot is quite different than that of the era when the adults of this report were children. We have shown that age 3 to 12 months is now the ideal age for elective repair of patients with tetralogy.[11] The adults in this series of late reoperations were much older at repair, 9.6 years, and more likely to have had a palliative operation prior to repair (44%) than is true of current practice.

The interval between repair and reoperation is long, on average 23.6 years. Hopefully current practice will both lengthen the interval to reoperation and decrease its prevalence. Meanwhile, we have shown that there is an increasing prevalence of adults presenting with late complications after previous repair in childhood, although of the total population at risk only 4.3% have come to reoperation. This population was repaired at a much older age than is true of current practice. Their median age at repair was 9.4 years, whereas our current age at repair is 8 months, and pre-repair palliation is rare.

The dominant problems in adults presenting late after tetralogy repair are pulmonary valve insufficiency and tachycardia, and we believe these are interrelated.

The timing of reintervention for pulmonary valve insufficiency is a difficult clinical decision. Most, if not all post-repair tetralogy patients, have some degree of pulmonary regurgitation. As Shimizaki has shown, patients with free pulmonary regurgitation from absent pulmonary valve and otherwise anatomically normal hearts do not become symptomatic until after the first 3 to 4 decades of life.[12] In this context, one might expect the post repair tetralogy patient to become symptomatic at a similar time, depending upon the degree of pulmonary regurgitation, the downstream pulmonary resistance, and the compliance of the right ventricle.[13] The timing of pulmonary valve replacement must be tempered by the inevitable failure of the prosthetic valve. Although older patient age and larger valve size are factors that improve valve durability, reintervention for prosthetic valve failure in this population is probable within 10 years in 15%, and increases rapidly beyond 10 years.[14] As Therrien has reported, pulmonary valve implantation may have been undertaken in our patients too late for functional recovery of the right ventricle.[15] However McLaughlin has shown that the majority of adults post tetralogy repair have stable right & left ventricular function.[16]

The decision to recommend pulmonary valve implantation is based upon development of symptoms, measurable limitation of exercise capacity, and objective evidence of deteriorating right heart function. The onset of atrial or ventricular arrhythmia often prompts surgical intervention, as it did in 40% of our patients.

Our data shows that reoperation is safe (1% operative risk of death) with good intermediate term survival (85% at 10 years) and a low rate of reintervention (four patients). The pulmonary valve prosthesis implanted in 90 patients has required replacement in two.

Ventricular tachycardia has been shown to be a risk factor for late sudden death after tetralogy repair.[17–19] Gatzoulis and colleagues reported that QRS width and its progressive increase after repair represent a risk factor for sudden death.[19] Thirty-three percent of our patients had VT prior to reoperation and its prevalence decreases following reintervention.[20,21] Whether cryoablation has an additional cardio-protective effect in terms of arrhythmia for repair of residual hemodynamic lesions is unclear. It is of note and reassuring that survival among those who had concomitant ablation for pre-existing arrhythmia was at least as good compared to patients without preoperative clinical arrhythmia. We have recently shown that pulmonary valve implantation alone stabilizes the QRS width and therefore acts as a risk modification procedure for VT and sudden cardiac death.[22]

Supraventricular tachycardia may also be improved by repair of the associated hemodynamic lesions, especially correction of tricuspid regurgitation. However, we know from the experience of older patients with an atrial septal defect and supraventricular tachycardia that the arrythmia tends to persist after an otherwise successful repair of the anatomic defect. Therefore we believe that ablative therapy for the atrial arrhythmia is an important adjunct to the reoperation. Further experience and longer follow-up is required to determine if ablation is efficacious.

Other lesions requiring reoperation are not common, and should decrease further because of continued improvement in operative techniques, including the important addition of quality control provided by intraoperative echocardiography. The development of aortic root dilation, leading to aortic regurgitation and aortic aneurysm is an interesting phenomenon. It has occurred in patients aged greater than 40 years who were repaired at an older age than the mean. It may be a late sequela of the aortic override, which is inherent in tetralogy. It may also be secondary to long-standing left heart volume overload due to late repair.

Conclusion

The adult with repaired tetralogy warrants ongoing life-long medical supervision to maintain their generally very favorable long-term outlook. In patients who develop late complications, surgical reintervention is safe, and provides long-term benefit.

References

1. Lillehei CW, Varco RL, Cohen M, et al. The first open heart repair of tetralogy of Fallot. A 26–31 year follow-up of 106 patients. *Ann Surg* 1986;294(4):490–502.
2. Roos-Hesselink J, Perlroth MG, McGhie J, et al. Atrial arrhythmias in adults after repair of tetralogy of Fallot. Correlations with clinical, exercise and echocardiographic findings. *Circulation* 1995;91:2214–2219.
3. Bricker JT. Sudden death and tetralogy of Fallot: Risks, markers and causes. *Circulation* 1995;92:162–163.
4. Jonsson H, Ivert T, Brodin LA, et al. Late sudden deaths after repair of tetralogy of Fallot. Electrocardiographic findings associated with survival. *Scand J Thorac Cardiovasc Surg* 1995;29:131–139.
5. Knott-Craig CJ, Elkins RC, Lane MM, et al. A 26-year experience with surgical management of tetralogy of Fallot: Risk analysis for mortality or late reintervention. *Ann Thorac Surg* 1998;66(2):506–511.

6. Castaneda AR, Freed MD, Williams RG, et al. Repair of tetralogy of Fallot in infancy. Early and late results. *J Thorac Cardiovasc Surg* 1977;74(3):372–381.

7. Deanfield JE. Adult congenital heart disease with special reference to the date on long-term follow-up of patients surviving to adulthood with or without surgical correction. *Eur Heart J* 1992;13:111–116.

8. Keith, Rowe, Vlad (eds), *Heart Disease in Infancy and Childhood,* 3rd edition, McMillan Publishing Inc. 1978.

9. Harrison DA, Harris L, Siu SC, et al. Sustained VT in adult patients late after repair of tetralogy of Fallot. *J Am Coll Cardiol* 1997;30:1368–1373.

10. Schaff HV, Dearani JA, Daly RC, et al. Cox-Maze procedure for atrial fibrillation: Mayo Clinic experience. *Sem Thorac Cardiovasc Surg* 2000;12:30–37.

11. Van Arsdell GS, Maharaj GS, Tom J, et al. What is the optimal age for repair of tetralogy of Fallot? *Circulation* 2000;102[suppl III]:III-123–129.

12. Kirklin JW, Blackstone EH, Jonas RA, et al. Morphologic and surgical determinants of outcome events after repair of tetralogy of Fallot and pulmonary stenosis. A two-institution study. *J Thorac Cardiovasc Surg* 1992;103:706–723.

13. Norgard G, Gatzoulis MA, Josen M, et al. Does restrictive right ventricular physiology in the early postoperative period predict subsequent right ventricular restriction after repair of tetralogy of Fallot? *Heart* 1998;79:481–484.

14. Caldarone CA, McCrindle BW, Van Arsdell GS, et al. Independent factors associated with longevity of prosthetic pulmonary valves. *J Thorac Cardiovasc Surg* 2000;120:1022–1031.

15. Therrien J, Siu SC, McLaughlin PR, et al. Pulmonary valve replacement in adults late after repair of tetralogy of Fallot: Are we operating too late? *J Am Coll Cardiol* 2000;36(5):1670–1675.

16. Gatzoulis MA, Elliott JT, Guru V, et al. Right and left ventricular function late after repair of tetralogy of Fallot: A longitudinal radionuclide angiographic study. *Am J Cardiol* 2000;86:1352–1357.

17. Gatzoulis MA, Till JA, Somerville J, et al. Mechano-electrical interaction in tetralogy of Fallot: QRS prolongation relates to right ventricular size and predicts malignant ventricular arrhythmias and sudden death. *Circulation* 1995;92:231–237.

18. Saul JP, Alexander ME. Preventing sudden death after repair of tetralogy of Fallot: Complex therapy for complex patients. *J Cardiovasc Electrophysiol* 1999;10:1271–1287.

19. Gatzoulis MA, Balaji S, Webber SA, et al. Risk factors for arrhythmia and sudden death in repaired tetralogy of Fallot: A multi-centre study. *Lancet* 2000;356:975–981.

20. Yemets IM, Williams WG, Webb GD, et al. Pulmonary valve replacement late after repair of tetralogy of Fallot. *Ann Thorac Surg* 1997;64:526–530.

21. Oechslin EN, Harrison DA, Harris L, et al. Reoperation in adults with repair of tetralogy of Fallot; Indications and outcomes. *J Thorac Cardiovasc Surg* 1999;118:245–251.

22. Therrien J, Siu S, Harris L, et al. Impact of pulmonary valve replacement on arrhythmia propensity late after repair of tetralogy of Fallot.*Circulation* 2001 (in press).

SUBJECT INDEX

Page numbers followed by "t" indicate tables.